Samuel '
The Ohio Sta

Working with People in Crisis

Theory and Practice

SECOND EDITION

Merrill, an imprint of
Macmillan Publishing Company
New York

Collier Macmillan Canada
Toronto

Maxwell Macmillan International Publishing Group
New York Oxford Singapore Sydney

To our children

Samuel, Pamela, and Mark

Macmillan Publishing Company
866 Third Avenue
New York, NY 10022

This book was set in Zapf.

Administrative Editor: Vicki Knight
Production Coordinator: Ben Shriver
Cover Designer: Cathy Watterson

Library of Congress Catalog Card Number: 86–62989
International Standard Book Number: 0–675–20701–0
Printed in the United States of America

5 6 7 8 9 — 91

Preface

This book is written for those who work with people in crisis, specifically students in any of the human services and beginning practitioners working in crisis intervention centers, suicide prevention centers, and mental health clinics. Its content and organization are based on my experience in working with people in crisis, teaching graduate students, and presenting workshops and seminars for people with varied educational backgrounds. Because of the variation in education and training of those working with people in crisis, fairly detailed knowledge of human behavior relevant to this process is presented. For some it may serve as a review; for others it may be new. Helping professionals should have a thorough understanding of human behavior before beginning to work with people in crisis.

Since the first edition of *Working with People in Crisis* was published in 1979, mental health professionals have used the crisis model in their service delivery system and have applied it to some problems not in the realm of the pure crisis model prior to 1980 (e.g., emergency medical services, spouse abuse, schools, hospitals, alcoholism). Although crisis theory was founded on a normative model of human reactions to threatening life events, its expanded use suggests that it is effective in the management of almost all acute distress.

The purpose of this book is to provide students and beginning practitioners with a crisis intervention model applicable to all people in crisis which at the same time makes individualized intervention possible. By relating crisis theory to the emotional and behavioral manifestations of people in crisis, a holistic approach to crisis intervention is presented. For example, a crisis condition can result from an overreaction to life-cycle events. A theoretical understanding of the life cycle can contribute to effective intervention.

Part I of this book explores theories of crisis and human behavior. Chapter 1 defines *crisis* and differentiates crises from everyday problems. Rather than briefly summarizing several theories of human behavior, Chapter 2 discusses only those characteristics manifested by those in crisis. The discussion of anxiety and depression has been expanded. Understanding these common crisis manifestations must transcend theoretical biases. Chapter 3 looks at the process of communication as it affects the interaction between client and therapist and the methods of intervention covered in later chapters. The discussion of communication is designed to give the therapist more conscious control of interviewing skills. Chapter 4 discusses the process and techniques of therapeutic intervention.

Part II integrates theory with practice. Chapter 5, based on foregoing theory, presents a model of intervention. It focuses on intervention methods and skill development. A discussion of assessment and evaluation helpful to graduate students and beginning practitioners has been added. The chapter also includes methods for group treatment of people in crisis. Chapter 6, which covers common crisis reactions, has been expanded to include separation and divorce and adolescent suicidal behavior. Chapter 7 discusses family and life-cycle crises.

The case illustrations included in this book are from many different records and settings. Names have been changed and situations disguised. If they seem recognizable, it is because of the universality of human experiences and reactions.

Many have contributed to the completion of this book. I would like to express my appreciation to Mrs. Nancy Graves, whose assistance was greatly appreciated; Dr. Rocco D'Angelo, Dr. Richard Bottcher, and Professor Milton Ain, whose support and encouragement will always be cherished; Dr. Robert C. Trojanowics, Michigan State University; and Drs. Gordon Hopper and Dominic Pellegrino, Iowa State University. Also, special thanks to Dr. Laura Epstein, the University of Chicago, and Dr. William H. Butterfield, Washington University, for their specific suggestions for improving the second edition.

Finally, I wish to thank my wife Clara and son Mark for their understanding support during the completion of this edition.

Samuel L. Dixon

Note to Instructors

Students learning to work effectively with people in crisis need to gain the skill and confidence that come from trying out the theory by applying it in practice situations. Role playing is a technique that allows students to practice their skills in class and receive feedback from instructor and fellow students. Students can play the roles of clients and workers in a variety of crisis situations, or actors and actresses may join the class to play out crises in which students can intervene. Scenarios can be drawn from case write-ups or from students' practice or practicum experience.

Contents

PART I

Conceptual Framework and Theoretical Base

PART I

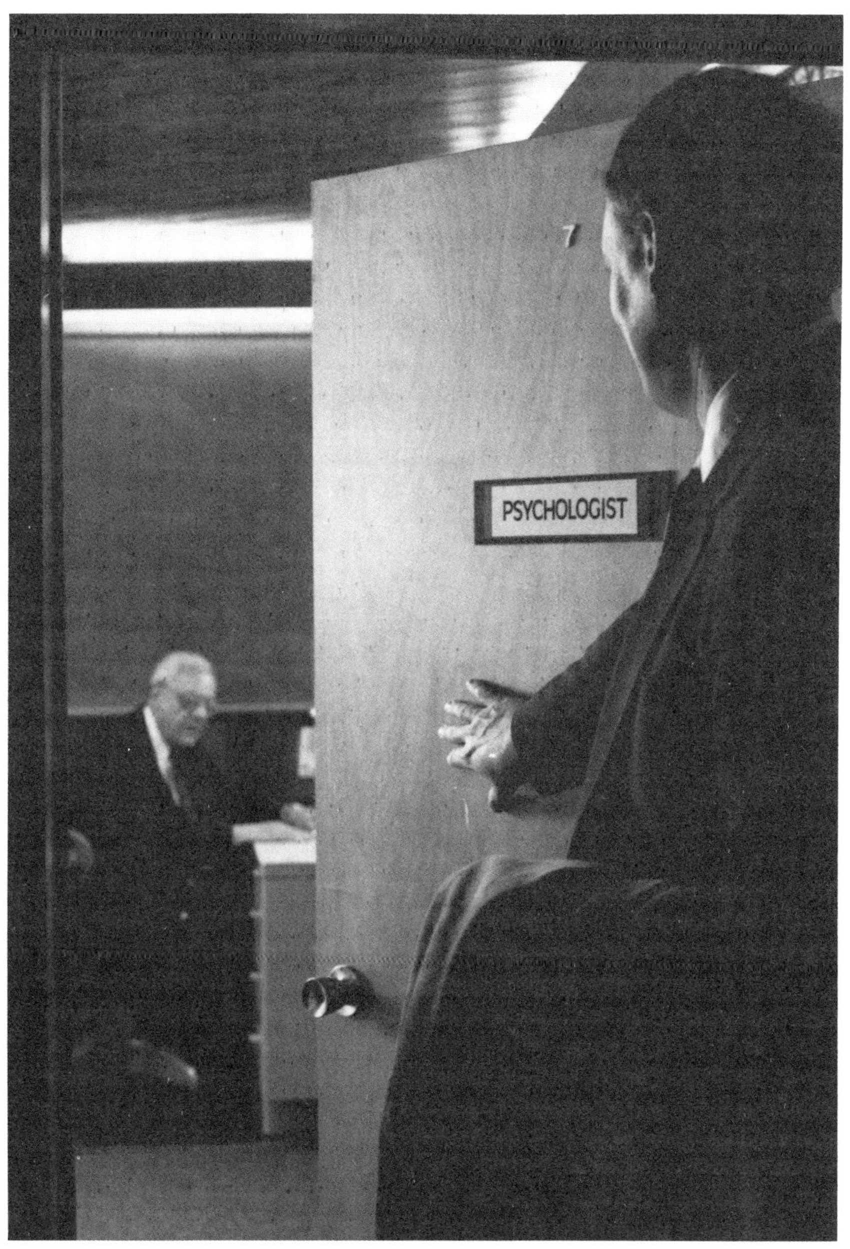

Conceptual Framework and Theoretical Base

1

Concept of Crisis

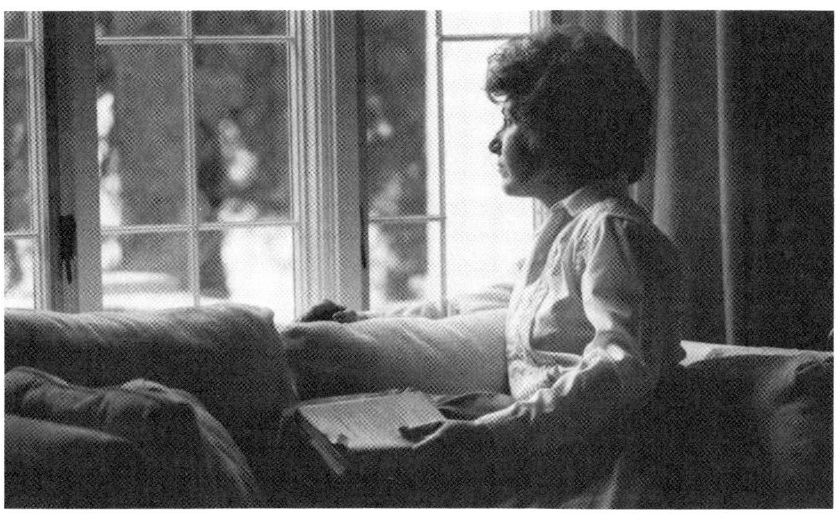

The ultimate goal of human beings is to achieve psychological comfort, a daily and continuous process. Fundamentally, people are prepared to pursue psychological comfort through the processes of biological development and socialization, from birth through adulthood. Love relationships, values, and other specific determiners of psychological comfort develop throughout the course of one's life. Systematic ways of feeling, perceiving, and behaving—in short, an integrated personality—result in each of us. Personality enables people to go about their daily activities unconsciously pursuing psychological comfort in a habituated and routine fashion. An integrated personality enables people to handle one eventuality after another as part of the course of living. There are times, however, when an event occurs that creates an insolvable problem that reduces the individual's ability to cope effectively because of a real or perceived danger. These are the conditions in which crises develop.

Crisis intervention techniques, skillfully applied, have been found to be effective with people in crisis regardless of their background or previous history. Originally, crisis theory was founded on the study of the behavior of people with no known history of psychopathology or mental illness; it was regarded as the study of adaptive and maladaptive reactions of "normal" people to accidental or natural catastrophes (Lindemann, 1944). Today, however, the crisis model is accepted by mental health professionals as a bona fide treatment modality for all types of individuals, thus making services available to more people than ever before. Let us look at several crisis situations as we begin to learn about the subject of crisis intervention.

Case Studies

Joanne, a 29-year-old woman who had been divorced twice, came to a crisis center after the sudden and unexpected death of her third husband. She felt she could no longer go on living. Although her first two marriages had ended in divorce, this third marriage, which lasted two years before her husband died, was one of unusual happiness. She credited a sense of personal salvation to this relationship. With her husband dead, Joanne was now extremely depressed. Before she came to the crisis center, she would leave the house only to go to the cemetery. Although she tried to forestall her progressive depression, she finally became deeply despairing and prepared to take her own life. Recognizing that her deceased husband would not want her to be that "weak," Joanne sought help at the crisis center. Following several sessions with the crisis therapist, her depression lifted and she returned to work and continued the normal grieving process without the extreme debilitation she had been feeling. About two months later, her father died, also suddenly and unexpectedly. Again she handled the situation alone as long as she could before returning to the crisis center. This time it was not the loss that overtaxed her strength, but the additional demands that her grieving mother now placed on her. A second therapist reached out to the mother and lightened the load on Joanne so that she could again function at her usual satisfactory level. In addition, the mother was helped through a stressful period, and a crisis was averted.

Martha, a 25-year-old married woman well along in her first pregnancy, came to a crisis center pleading for relief from tormenting fears. She was afraid that she was going to die and that her unborn child would be born deformed or handicapped. These suspicions made her afraid that she was going to lose her mind. The terrifying feelings had started immediately after she learned she was pregnant.

Richard, a 37-year-old executive, called a crisis center because he felt overwhelmed by feelings of rage, frustration, disappointment, and resentment. His emotions were keeping him from carrying out his normal responsibilities. These feelings had begun shortly after he was passed over for a higher position that he felt he deserved because of his experience and ability. The job was given to a less experienced, less capable man. Richard expressed feelings of personal failure and dejection. He said that he was so hurt by this rejection he could not bear the pain. It was a violent attack on his self-esteem and pride.

Joanne, Martha, and Richard each went through a crisis—an increasingly common occurrence. Probably no subject of study is more applicable today than the study of crisis. The combination of human nature and the hazardous, uncertain, and anxiety-ridden world we live in increases the likelihood that everyone will face some situation that is potentially crisis producing. However, crisis is not new; it has always been a part of the human existence.

In fact, human beings are born in a state of crisis—the birth trauma. From the very moment of birth, many of our efforts are intended to avoid crisis. Because neither human nature nor the external environment allows the needs, desires, and goals of any one person to be achieved unequivocally, people inevitably experience stress (Erikson, 1959). But we also have the capacity to adapt to our environment so that we pursue goals that fit our society, goals that are socially determined. To this end we develop habitual patterns of adaptation as we grow up and are socialized into our culture. Habitual patterns of adaptation as used here means the human being's actions and reactions. It refers to a person's customary ways of functioning, including goals and values. It includes the ways in which people maintain control of themselves in relation to the environment. It is synonymous with personality.

We go along in our lives taking for granted our ability to respond to the world and to solve problems, until something happens to interfere. Upsetting events such as natural catastrophies, illnesses, separations, deaths, and personal losses have always been part of living. But there used to be more extended family and close friends to step in and help an individual with a problem.

The systematic approach by professionals to helping people in crisis is relatively new. Its origin is credited to Lindemann (1944) and Caplan (1964). Since these two pioneers wrote the initial descriptions of the process, crisis intervention has grown enormously as a treatment modality. Its growth is attributed to several factors. First, there has been an increase in public acceptance of the idea of turning to professionals for help. In addition, there seem to be more potentially crisis-producing events than ever: conflicts over desegregation, problems of intimacy, marriage and divorce, changing social roles, unemployment, and increased crimes all can lead to a personal crisis. And we place greater emphasis today on the individual's "right" to achieve a personal goal. We are increasingly competitive; we face more open conflict than ever before and, hence, greater tension and stress. At the same time we are more mobile. Few of us live in large, supportive, extended families; many of us are geographically separated from family and close, lifelong friends to whom we can turn for emotional support and help. A second reason for the popularity of crisis intervention therapy was proposed by Lindemann and Caplan: we have come to see that intervention at the point of crisis can prevent the development of maladaptive patterns of behavior or serious mental breakdown and might even improve personality. Third, crisis intervention techniques, skillfully applied, have been found to be effective not just with people in crisis, but with all acutely distressed people, regardless of their background or previous history. This claim is now accepted by mental health professionals whose traditional interest was in psychopathology.

CRISIS THEORY

Crisis theory draws from a number of human behavior or personality theories, including ego psychology, learning theory, existentialism, and system theory. The theory or theories an individual applies when dealing with people in crisis must include in its concepts and definitions those aspects of human behavior universally manifested by those in crisis. Crisis theory, as used in this book, is based on a holistic concept of personality, where personality is seen as always evolving through experience. The accumulated life experiences, from birth through adulthood, result in an organized psychic system. Each individual's psychic system is dynamic; it is influenced by biological, psychological, and sociological experiences and events. The psychic system could also be called the *ego*, the *self*, or simply a set of learned patterns of thinking and behaving that are the result of the socialization process. This concept implies the influence and inseparable relationship between the human being and the environment.

To understand this better, let us briefly look at the development of the psychic system (see also chapter 2). Human infants are born helpless but with a set of biological reflexes that help them survive by communicating their needs to a parent or other caretaker. Most infants also have capacities that ultimately will let them function independently. The child's ability to function independently grows according to his or her individual maturational and developmental schedule. But not only do human infants need another person to take care of basic survival needs, they also need someone to stimulate their innate capacities for independent social functioning. Furthermore, the direction of individual development is also determined by the social environment. In sum, the human being is biologically endowed to function independently, but the specific way any individual functions is determined by psychosocial experiences within the specific environment.

The human capacities for adaptation—perception, memory, intelligence, mobility, emotions, consciousness, and purpose—enable individuals to retain and recall experiences so that they can organize their emotions and intellect into specific and habitual patterns of social functioning. In this regard, each person brings to each new situation a set of responses, needs, feelings, attitudes, values, and expectations, all the result of unique life experiences that are both personal and interpersonal. The psychic system, values, and goals of every person are different from those of every other person because life experiences, social environments, and ways of learning are different. Thus each person's perceptions, psychic reality, and reactions to various stimuli and events also differ. Any two people, even identical twins, will experience the same situation differently.

Satisfying Needs

The foundation stimulus of all human behavior is survival (Hartmann, 1958). If life is endangered, all other needs pale in comparison, and the degree of satisfaction of survival needs influences the degree to which a person is able to concentrate on psychosocially determined needs. In other words, the degree to which people can concentrate on higher processes is determined in part by whether they must worry about survival. If survival is threatened, even a well-adjusted person experiences a crisis, and *the threat does not have to be real in fact but only perceived as real.*

When survival is not threatened, psychosocially determined needs are more important. They can, and often do, assume a value as high as that of survival. The case of Joanne, Martha, and Richard illustrate how important psychological needs can become.

When the human being's survival needs are adequately satisfied, the process of qualitative psychic development can take place. Consequently, parents and significant others are very important in the functioning of the child's psychic system. As infants mature, they learn quickly that parents are the source of satisfaction of their survival needs; dependence on parents produces a life and death attachment. As infants grow, they begin to recognize that to maintain parental love, affection, and protection, parents must be pleased. Thus the child's psychosocial needs such as love, respect, recognition, and security assume primary importance when the child is confident that survival needs will be satisfied. In effect, survival needs become secondary until the child perceives them to be threatened. Another need that develops as survival and love needs are met is the need for achievement or self-fulfillment. This drive develops with age and experience. By the time people reach adulthood, they have accumulated a unique psychic system that reflects all perceptions of self and the environment.

This idiosyncratic process creates the variations we see in people's behavior. Most important, each individual evolves a system for functioning in habitual ways to meet personal needs and goals, to meet the demands and limitations of the social environment, and to resolve everyday problems. In general, this personal system keeps people in relative equilibrium and enables them to restore equilibrium when it is upset.

Because there are always many internal and external stimuli in people's lives, temporary disequilibrium or upset is common enough that it can be regarded as part of the human condition. To react to conflicting stimuli, an individual simply uses habitual patterns of adaptation to restore equilibrium, then sets about resolving the next conflict or meeting the next need. Each person learns techniques for coping with stress that allow him or her to carry out daily responsibilities while attempting to maintain internal constancy.

The process of maintaining psychic equilibrium is called homeostasis. It is a process that is so much a part of life that it is probably taken for granted. Many people are unaware of the ways in which they attempt to maintain homeostasis. But just ask yourself what do you do most often when you are angry? When you are depressed? How do you get over upsetting feelings? Whatever you do is the way you restore and maintain equilibrium.

Restoring equilibrium while satisfying various needs and reacting to conflicting stimuli is the basis of all social functioning. The degree to which a person is successful in this process is a very important measure of social functioning, since emotional upset interferes with effectiveness. Because there is so much to react to, most people develop patterns that let them react to a whole class of things in similar ways. These familiar patterns help keep emotional upset to manageable proportions. When a person cannot keep emotional upset manageable, when none of the usual ways of responding works, two conditions can result: (a) a crisis that can be successfully resolved or (b) an unresolved crisis that will lead to the development of new, maladaptive patterns.

A human being's emotional state is constantly changing. In graphic terms we can think of a perfect emotional life with no stress as a straight line. As shown in Figure 1.1, we would expect that most people would waver above and below the baseline most of the time. We can call this state *average expectable behavior* (term adapted from Hartmann [1958], Concept of Average Expectable Environment). The term *average expectable behavior* is a more accurate term than *normal,* as many deviations from average are "normal." Note that the length of time that a person is at a steady state, exactly on the baseline, is very short.

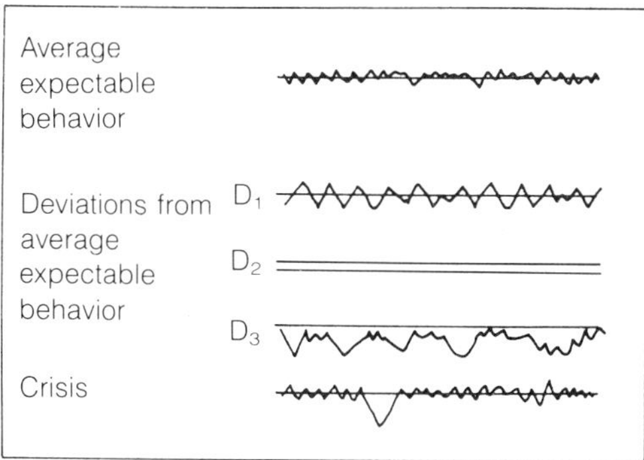

FIGURE 1.1 Degrees of social functioning.

Some people's behavior deviates from average expectable behavior to such an extent that they would traditionally be thought to show clinical syndromes. D_1 falls within the clinical syndrome or diagnostic category commonly called anxiety disorders, D_2 points to personality disorders, and D_3 to psychoses (see DSM III, *Diagnostic and Statistical Manual,* American Psychiatric Association, 1980).

Historically, these terms have been used to describe the varying degrees of psychopathology, sometimes called mental illness, and often referred to in psychology books as abnormal psychology. The common basis of psychopathology is faulty personality development. In simple terms this means that the socialization process (i.e., the satisfaction of needs for love, security, acceptance, recognition, and guidance in a social environment responsible for the nature of interpersonal relationships and opportunities for self-fulfillment) was not conducive to the development of a psychic system that enables the individual to satisfy personal needs and goals within the limitations, expectations, and demands of the social environment. Consequently, patterns of thinking, feeling, and behaving characteristic of the clinical syndromes are developed as a compromise effort to meet personal and common human needs, to adapt to the social environment (regardless of how maladaptive), and most important, to prevent total personality disintegration. It should be remembered that although patterns of human behavior can be identified and classified, behavior is best represented by the concept of a continuum. This means that all human beings experience the same feelings and behavior; the difference is in quantity, not in kind. In other words, everyone at some time or another will experience feelings or exhibit behavior characteristic of the clinical syndromes. However, to temporarily experience such behavior is not the same as being diagnosed as having an anxiety disorder, personality disorder, or psychosis. To merit that diagnosis means that the person's *habitual* patterns of behavior are characterized by such a clinical syndrome. Of the clinical syndromes, the anxiety disorders are the least severe. They are characterized by such habitual (*not* transitory) patterns of behavior as anxiety states, phobias, or obsessive-compulsive behaviors.

Personality disorders are more severe than anxiety disorders but not as severe as psychoses. Personality disorders are characterized by patterns of maladaptive behavior such as acting out, impulsiveness, irresponsibility, or antisocial behavior. Psychoses, the most severe, are characterized by breaks with reality and an almost total psychic or personality disintegration, usually manifested by delusions and hallucinations. Actively psychotic individuals generally require hospitalization. The term *mentally ill* is more appropriately used for those experiencing psychoses than other clinical syndromes. It should be clear that a clinical syndrome's degree of interference with living varies from person to person, depending on the nature of the social environment and the existence of certain events. Some social environments prevent potential psychotic breakdowns and, conversely, others contribute to psychotic breakdowns.

With this understanding of the clinical syndromes, let us return to Figure 1.1. We can see that the deviations from the solid line are greater and last longer than deviations in average expectable behavior.

In contrast, the crisis behavior line does not vary much from that of average expectable behavior until the occurrence of the event precipitating the crisis. At this point the emotional state drops far below the baseline. But once the crisis has passed, the graph returns to the average expectable behavior level.

WHAT IS A CRISIS?

Although the word *crisis* is extensively used, it is often misunderstood. Most people associate crisis with a temporary state of upset that exists while a problem is being solved. People say such things as, "I had a crisis this morning," or "Bob is really upset." But as we have seen, being upset is an integral part of daily living. We deal with everyday stress with habitual patterns of adaptation and restore our ability to maintain with some variability our usual level of social functioning. A true crisis occurs when excessive emotionality prevents individuals from solving a problem by the usual problem-solving methods. As a consequence, personal upset increases until it is impossible to function as efficiently as before the problem occurred.

A true crisis is more than a temporary state of upset; it is an inability to function effectively as a consequence of the emotional turmoil. A person experiencing a real crisis is unable to solve the problem effectively. If a person can effectively solve a problem even though he or she is upset, then that individual is not in crisis but is engaging in the common problems of living. It is personality disorganization and ineffective problem-solving that constitutes a crisis condition. Hence, we can define a crisis as a functionally debilitating emotional state resulting from the individual's reaction to some event perceived to be so dangerous that it leaves him or her feeling helpless and unable to cope effectively by usual methods. Let us look at the four major elements of this definition.

Precipitating Event

Each human being's capacity to tolerate stress and the pressures of life is finite and idiosyncratic. Under certain conditions or situations, everyone has a breaking point at which habitual patterns of adaptation and problem-solving methods are no longer effective in maintaining the usual degree of social functioning. A precipitating event in a crisis situation is always related to a perceived threat to survival or bodily integrity or to one or more psychosocial needs that have assumed a primary value. Consequently, the idiosyncratic meaning of the precipitating event can only be found in the person's own reality, which houses his or her personal feelings, goals, expectations, and values, all determined by specific life experiences.

A specific event in some form almost always precipitates a crisis, even if the individual cannot readily identify the event. The cognitive processes of a person in crisis may be impaired to the point that the person is not aware of or cannot remember the precipitating event. Furthermore, the precipitating event could have occurred several weeks before the person becomes functionally impaired. It is not unusual for a person who is already feeling overwhelmed to be unable to sort out the first link in this chainlike process. The search for a precipitating event, when it is not obvious, is a very important therapeutic process. Sometimes you may need to look at the events of several preceding weeks, although the precipitating event can usually be found to have occurred within two weeks of the crisis. As Bloom (1965) concludes:

> The single most contributory variable involved in the crisis judgment in the present sample appears to be the experience of a precipitating event. On this basis, one could simply define the crisis state as inevitably following certain specified events.

If the functional debilitation is *not* related to a specific event, the excessive emotional response is probably a part of some clinical disorder. Bloom (1965) found that clinical experts reached greater agreement in defining a crisis when there was a known precipitating event than when it was unknown. Farberow (1967) believes that if all the components of a crisis are present except the known precipitating event, the person is probably experiencing psychiatric disorder. (But individuals with psychiatric disorders also develop crises.)

The idea of a precipitating event is central in the development of the theory of crisis, beginning with Lindemann (1944), who studied people's reactions to a known catastrophic event, the Coconut Grove nightclub fire in Boston. His work led to the recognition that any event that threatens human survival or significant needs or values can precipitate a state of crisis in any person, regardless of the person's psychological history. The theory has led to the idea that a crisis is a turning point that represents both a danger and an opportunity (Morley, 1970). The danger is that the person who does not resolve the crisis will develop a clinical syndrome; the opportunity is for emotional growth as a result of learning from the experience.

To understand how such diverse events as divorce, pregnancy, or retirement can precipitate a crisis, the nature of the event and its significance and meaning to the individual must be understood in the context of both past and present experiences.

For example, Mary, age 41, was told by her husband of 25 years that he wanted a divorce. The crisis resulted from Mary's disappointed expectations that she would be married forever, from her feelings that she was not good enough to keep her husband and that she was incapable of taking care of herself in spite of the fact that she had worked for more than 23 years of her married life and currently earned an adequate salary. Rapoport (1965) states that an initial blow can be perceived as (a) a threat to either instinctual needs or to the sense of physical and emotional integrity; (b) loss of a person, an ability, or a capability; or (c) a challenge that threatens to overtax an individual's capacities. Mary's perception of this event met all three criteria. It is essential to find out what the event means to the individual, how it is perceived to be a threat, and how and why it is interpreted as it is. The real meaning of the event can be found in either present or past life experiences. In Mary's case, understanding the past is the key to understanding her crisis. She grew up with a very disturbed mother who made her feel extremely insecure and distrustful. She married her husband out of a need for security, sensing his strong need to take care of her. He was her refuge from a very dangerous world.

To sum up, then, the existence of a visible precipitating event is one of the most salient characteristics of a crisis and one that generally distinguishes it from psychopathology. The precipitating event is an occurrence perceived by an individual to be a grave threat. To an observer, the event may appear to be insignificant, but to the person in crisis it is very serious. The interpretations of the event are laden with personal meaning based on either past or present experiences.

Perceived Meaning

Again, a crisis is a subjective state; it is the personal meaning attributed to the precipitating event that causes the person's excessive emotional state. While pregnancy precipitated a crisis for Martha, it does not for most women. In simple terms, a crisis is not caused by an event itself but is a reaction to an event. Reaction is determined by perceptual interpretation and meaning. Events have only the meaning given to them by the individual; event, perception, interpretation, and reactions cause crisis. Crisis conditions are subjectively and individually determined. Hence a crisis can only be understood from the frame of reference of the individual experiencing it.

Ineffective Problem-Solving Methods

Crises are usually precipitated by events so common that they can potentially happen to everyone. Although there are some events so universally significant that a crisis condition is expected, not all such events produce crises. Once a significant event occurs, everyone initially attempts to deal with it by applying their usual methods of problem solving. The difference between the person who develops a crisis and one who does not is related to the personal interpretation of the meaning of that event. The individual who develops a crisis interprets the meaning of the event as lying beyond the capacity of his or her usual coping methods and patterns of adaptation. As the individual continues making ineffective attempts to solve the problem created by the precipitating event, regression occurs as emotionalism increases. As cognitive functioning fails and emotionalism dominates one's efforts, the individual tends to resort more frequently to inappropriate methods, thus making his or her efforts even more ineffective. Emotionalism increases progressively as ineffectiveness increases. As Caplan (1961) states:

> When a person faces an obstacle to important life goals . . . [that is] for a time insurmountable through the utilization of customary methods of problem solving [a] period of disorganization ensues, a period of upset, during which many abortive attempts at solution are made.

Caplan (1964) describes the progressive nature of a crisis as follows:

1. There is an initial rise of tension from the impact of an external event, which in turn initiates habitual "problem-solving responses."
2. The lack of success of these problem solving responses, plus the continued impact of the stimulus event, further increases tension, feelings of upset, and ineffectuality.
3. As the tension increases, other problem-solving resources are mobilized. At this point, the crisis may be arrested by any of the following: reduction of the external threat, success of new coping strategies,

redefinition of the problem, or the giving up of tightly held but unobtainable goals.
4. If more of these occurs, however, the tension mounts to a breaking point, resulting in severe emotional disorganization.

The important point is that the person in crisis will feel unable to deal effectively with the problem. The person who is not in crisis may be very upset but is able to deal effectively with the problem. But for the individual in crisis the real or subjectively perceived threat is so significant that the inability to solve the problem will result in dire consequences. Anticipation of those consequences further increases the emotionality and feelings of helplessness.

So when habitual patterns of adaptation and coping mechanisms are no longer effective and emotionalism dominates the individual's behavior, the condition is a crisis. The emotional condition *is* the crisis which reduces the individual's cognitive functioning (Taplin, 1971). This point is central to the treatment of a person in crisis and will be elaborated on in Part II.

Functionally Debilitating Emotional State

The excessiveness of the response separates the individual in crisis from the temporarily upset person involved in solving a problem. For example, if a mechanical system malfunctioned during a space flight, the astronauts would probably become upset; that is, they would feel fear or anxiety, perspire profusely, and have increased heart palpitations. However, if the astronauts were still able to take the necessary measures to correct the situation and to make reasonable decisions in an effort to solve the problem, they would not be in crisis. On the other hand, if their emotional reaction was so excessive that they could not remember what to do and could not make reasonable decisions, they would be in crisis.

A person in crisis is unable to reason effectively. Thinking capacity is overwhelmed by the emotional response. Now the occurrence of some events in life are so provocative that the appropriate emotional response can be of crisis proportions and not be abnormal, depending on the duration. For instance, the death of a loved one is so crucial that the person who does not feel extreme grief for a time can be in more serious trouble than someone making an excessive response.

IDENTIFYING A PERSON IN CRISIS

Since a state of upset is a common occurrence for everyone at some time in their lives, how do we know when a person is in crisis? There are several characteristics that we initially recognize to differentiate a person in crisis from the person who is merely upset.

First, there is generally the event perceived to have precipitated the crisis. Examples, some of which we've already touched on, include marital or family separation, divorce, death of a loved one, or loss of a beloved home. It may be a loss or threatened loss of self-esteem, identity, self-concept, status, or position. The birth of a child, healthy or defective, or a change in occupation can precipitate a crisis, as can a loss or perceived loss of a material possession or economic and social achievement, for example, a major drop in the value of a stock holding. Certain critical points in the life cycle can precipitate a crisis, such as the beginning of adolescence or birth of a first grandchild. Again, understanding the precipitating event is the key to understanding the person in crisis. Tables 1.1 and 1.2 show Morrice's (1976) compilation of common precipitating events from 266 consecutive admissions to the Ross Clinic in Aberdeen, Scotland, and from 85 emergency services in the United States.

A second characteristic is that the person in crisis experiences an overwhelming degree of emotionality (i.e., anxiety, depression, guilt, shame, etc.) which makes him or her feel helpless and unable to behave effectively. This symptom has already been mentioned; different manifestations of these emotions are discussed in chapter 2. An unusual degree of personality disorganization and impaired social functioning results from this excessive emotionality. Because the individual's habitual patterns of adaptation are not effective, they are abandoned. The ability to think and reason logically is impaired, and so the individual may turn from external reality toward the self. Because the individual feels confused and unable to cope with the situation at this time, he or she is most accessible to help. He or she is generally not defensive, self-protective, or mistrustful. This period of heightened disorganization

TABLE 1.1 *All crises identified in 266 admissions to day hospital*

Nature of crisis	*Number*	*Percent*
Interpersonal difficulty in family	249	51
Antisocial behavior	30	6
Work problem	110	22
Financial problem	35	7
Physical illness	22	4
Bereavement	27	6
Accident	4	1
Pregnancy	8	2
Other	5	1
TOTAL	490	100

TABLE 1.2 *Nature of problems cited by 85 emergency services in United States*

Nature of Problem	*Incidence*
Family conflict including marital discord and impending divorce	51
Excessive use of alcohol	27
Problems relating to job or income	19
Bereavement or grief reaction	16
Exacerbation of chronic mental illness	12
Problems of adolescence	6
Problems of old age	5
School problems	4
Medical illness	4
Separation from familiar environment	3
Homosexual panic	3
Legal charges	2
Postpartum depression	2
Postoperative reaction	2

usually lasts only a short while. It is the point for immediate and rapid intervention. Occasionally, however, by the time the professional person sees the individual in crisis, the emotionalism has been suppressed or retarded and what is manifested are feelings of helplessness, inadequacy, exhaustion, or physical symptoms. Even when emotionalism is not manifested in some form, it resides within the individual and should become a major focus, a point that will be discussed later.

A third characteristic, again previously touched on, is the ineffectiveness of habitual patterns of problem solving and coping methods. This condition alone increases emotionalism and the feeling of helplessness. The individual's patterns of adaptation and problem-solving methods generally have been effective for a number of years. It is easy to understand the emotional state produced by the ineffectiveness of adaptive patterns that have been relatively effective until the crisis point for the person who does not know why they are no longer effective.

A fourth characteristic of a crisis is that it is time-limited. Caplan (1964) held that crises usually can be resolved within four to six weeks. Actually, some crises can be resolved in four to six weeks while others require a longer period of time. It should be noted that what is resolved in such a short period of time is some of the emotional debilitation and subjective discomfort; the *effects* of the crisis may last longer. In some cases, such as grief and bereavement crises, the effect may last for years and never be completely resolved. Therapists have to decide whether the effects of the crisis require continued treatment beyond the temporal nature of the crisis.

CAUSES OF CRISIS

Crisis theory assumes that social functioning is a continuous effort to maintain and restore equilibrium as one is exposed to potentially upsetting problems of living and pursuing goals. Each person maintains psychic equilibrium through individual adaptive patterns and coping mechanisms. Since everyone is exposed to potentially crisis-producing events, an important question is why a certain event causes a crisis for some people and not for others. We know that the same event that causes a crisis for one person may be perceived by another as a challenge to be overcome. *The cause of a crisis is the significance of the event to the person involved.* Hence the basis for understanding and helping a person in crisis is through his or her subjective frame of reference or psychic reality. It is Martha's personal interpretation of pregnancy that represents a danger. It is Richard's reaction to being passed over that renders his habitual patterns of adaptation ineffective, creating the feeling of helplessness.

The next question is what causes the person in crisis to interpret the event as he or she does. The precipitating event is always associated with some kind of internal experience. It may not be the strength of the personality that determines whether a person develops a crisis. Rather, the determining factor may be whether an event is significant enough to the individual and occurs at a time when he or she is vulnerable. Another factor is the strength of the individual's defenses against the particular feelings brought on by the precipitating event. Most reactions to crisis-producing events involve anxiety or depression or their derivatives. (Suicide and homicide are derivations of anxiety or depression.) Understanding these two universal emotions can be the key to understanding the meaning of the precipitating event for the person in crisis. They are discussed in depth in chapter 2.

CRISIS THERAPY VERSUS TRADITIONAL PSYCHOTHERAPY

At this point, distinction needs to be made between crisis therapy and traditional psychotherapy. (No significant *qualitative* difference is intended by the use of the words *crisis therapy and psychotherapy,* however. Crisis therapy is also psychotherapy.)

As Jacobson (1970) states:

> The [crisis] therapist must be clear that he is dealing with a self-contained modality with its own particular characteristics. This modality in no way substitutes for other forms of psychotherapy, whether of immediate length or long-term, nor does it eliminate the need in some cases for full or partial

hospitalization. It is one string in the therapeutic bow; but a string with its own particular and unique qualities.

There are, however, several differences between crisis therapy and other therapies. First, crisis theory does not assume psychopathology or an underlying intrapsychic conflict, although persons with these problems can experience crisis. The spectrum of "normal" human behavior is broad enough to allow individuals with all sorts of other difficulties to benefit at times from short-term crisis therapy.

The purpose of crisis therapy is to return the person to his or her previous level of social functioning. For example, Marianne, a young divorcee who had been progressing well in psychotherapy, experienced a crisis when her 10-year-old son Dan demanded to leave her to live with his father and started to make the arrangements. Marianne presented the classic symptoms of a person in crisis; the crisis had to be resolved before she could return to her previous level of functioning and make further progress in her psychotherapy.

A related question is whether crisis therapy treats a person's underlying conflicts. Although everyone has these conflicts (Erikson, 1959; Hartmann, 1958), they are not significant except as they relate specifically to the treatment process. An individual may have reactivated an underlying conflict in the effort to resolve the current crisis. If the problem does not respond to crisis intervention and continues to influence the person's social functioning, more traditional psychotherapy is probably indicated.

The second distinction between crisis therapy and traditional psychotherapy is the existence of a real precipitating event that unites the individual's internal and external worlds. Crisis theory assumes that the individual has no uncommon weakness in his or her general ability to adapt to life. Rather, it is the reaction to an event that causes a *temporary* social dysfunctioning, the outcome of which is significant to future social functioning.

A third distinction between crisis therapy and traditional psychotherapy is that the former is practiced in a variety of places and settings, for example, emergency rooms of hospitals, the client's home, or on the street, as well as offices of mental health clinics and counseling and crisis centers. Regardless of the setting, the practice of crisis therapy is basically the same.

A final distinction is the temporal nature of a crisis. By definition most crises can be resolved in less than seven weeks, although the effects may last longer. Problems requiring traditional intervention usually take considerably longer to resolve or even to achieve a given level of improvement.

GOALS OF CRISIS THERAPY

The goals of crisis therapy are the resolution of the individual's crisis, a change in perception of danger, and the restoration of social functioning to at least the precrisis level. As Paul (1966) states:

> In reversing the decompensation and restoring emotional equilibrium, we aim to strengthen the client's resources, to give him not only symptom relief, but also symptom control, social control, and some degree of insight.

For the individual who understands the theory of crisis, these are reasonably achievable goals compared with other psychotherapeutic efforts. The person in crisis is more amenable to help than at any other time in life. The feelings of helplessness make the person receptive to help; they increase the desire to learn to cope with a new situation. At the same time, the situation is delicate and requires special skills that traditional therapies may not require. Perhaps the first is the ability to intervene at a time when not much information can easily be acquired. The therapist also needs to be able to quickly establish a tentative formulation of the client's condition. Second, the therapist must often be able to define the precipitating event and its meaning for the client. Third, the therapist is often much more active and involved than traditional therapists. Fourth, the therapist must be able to elicit powerful and painful feelings such as the reactions a client has to impending death. Fifth, and closely related, is the capacity of the therapist to tolerate painful emotions in others, to tolerate human suffering. Sixth, the therapist must be willing to assume responsibility for others. Finally, the therapist must have confidence in his or her ability to help a person in crisis. Goldstein (1962) found that the therapist's self-confidence has a significant impact on the client's improvement. In effect, the crisis therapist must have the ability to quickly evaluate, teach, and facilitate problem resolutions. A sound theoretical understanding of how people behave is essential if you are to be effective with people in crisis. Some basic ways in which people behave are discussed in chapter 2.

STRESS AND CRISIS

Recently, the concept of stress has been associated with crisis. The two terms are often used interchangeably; whether stress and crisis are the same depends upon how the terms are used. Stress and crisis are synonymous if stress is conceived as a reaction to a life event (called the stressor) (Dohrenwend and Dohrenwend, 1981), and the other characteristics of a crisis are present. However, stress and crisis are different if stress is viewed as a process. In the latter case, stress is viewed as a strain under severe circumstances, adverse conditions, or important situations. For example, working as a crisis therapist or working with the pressure of meeting deadlines can be stressful. That is, trying to meet some goal or accomplish some task under pressure is stressful, but it is not a crisis.

Pressure situations produce stress because extraordinary energy is required to accomplish this goal. In such situations, stress can produce both psychological and physiological changes. Selye (1956) described three stages of stress response that constitute a general adaptation syndrome (GAS): alarm, resistance, and exhaustion (see table 1.3). The thought of failure also adds pressure, making the situation stressful. Although the reaction to failure under a stressful condition can be a crisis, there are several important differences between stress and crisis: (a) people live and work under stress for years, thus making it a way of life (e.g., air traffic controllers); (b) stress is usually clearly perceived (e.g., trying to accomplish a goal by a given date); and (c) stressful situations can be either pleasurable and satisfying or painful (e.g., the stress of trying to meet a United Way fund-raising goal). In crisis, the event is generally unexpected, the adverse reaction is acute, temporal in nature, and emotionally debilitating. It should be noted, however, that after the occurrence of the event, one experiences stress when trying to resolve the problem leading up to the crisis condition.

EMERGENCY AND CRISIS

Emergencies and crises are generally considered in tandem. However, there are some notable differences between the two. An emergency is a crisis, but a crisis may not be an emergency. An emergency is a situation that poses an immediate real danger to the life of the individual or others, and direct action must be taken immediately: a knife wound, a heart attack, a drug overdose, a full blown psychosis, a suicide attempt. Although emergencies respond to crisis intervention theory and technique, they may not be amenable to the whole process of crisis intervention. The immediate task is generally to save the person's life, which

TABLE 1.3 *Selye's General Adaptation Syndrome (GAS)*

Stage	*Characteristic Response*
Alarm	Stress activates the mobilization of adaptive mechanism.
Resistance	Stress requires sustaining high-level use of adaptive mechanism.
Exhaustion	Stress depletes mechanisms through prolonged use.

may take less than six weeks or it may take more. Some hospitals may not assume responsibility beyond saving the individual's life.

SUMMARY

This chapter emphasizes the universality of human crises and presents a conceptual frame of reference for understanding people in crisis. At this point you should understand the basic premise of crisis theory, what a crisis is, and how it differs from common problems of living. Of particular importance, you should be able to identify the characteristics of a person in crisis and should understand why one person develops a crisis and another does not. The differences between crisis intervention and traditional psychotherapy are also discussed.

REFERENCES

American Psychiatric Association. (1980). *Diagnostic and statistical manual of mental disorders* (DSM III) (3rd ed.). Washington, D.C.: Author.

Bloom, B. L. (1965). Definitional aspects of the crisis concept. In H. J. Parad (Ed.), *Crisis intervention: Selected readings.* (pp. 303–311). New York: Family Service Association of America.

Caplan, G. (1961). *An approach to community mental health.* New York: Grune & Stratton.

Caplan, G. (1964). *Principles of preventive psychiatry.* New York: Basic Books.

Dohrenwend, S., & Dohrenwend, B. P. (1981). *Stressful life events and their contexts.* New York: Prodist.

Erikson, E. H. (1959). Growth and crises of the health personality. In Identity and the life cycle: Selected papers. [Monograph]. *Psychological Issues, 1*(1), 50–100.

Farberow, N. L. (1967). Crisis, disaster and suicide: Theory and therapy. In E. S. Shneidman (Ed.), *Essays in self-destruction.* New York: Science House.

Goldstein, A. P. (1962). *Therapist-patient expectations in psychotherapy.* New York: Macmillan.

Hartmann, H. (1958). Ego psychology and the problem of adaptation. [Monograph Series, No. 1]. *Journal of the American Psychoanalytic Association.*

Jacobson, G. F. (1970) Crisis intervention from the viewpoint of the mental health professional. *Pastoral Psychology, 21*(203), 21–28.

Lindemann, E. (1965). Symptomatology and management of acute grief. In H. J. Parad (Ed.), *Crisis intervention: Selected readings.* (pp. 7–21). (Reprinted from *American Journal of Psychiatry,* 1944, *101*)

Morley, W. E. (1970). Theory of crisis intervention. *Pastoral Psychology, 21*(203), 14–20.

Morrice, J. K. W. (1976). *Crisis intervention: Studies in community care.* Oxford, England: Pergamon Press.

Paul, L. (1966). Crisis intervention. *Mental Hygiene, 50*(1), 141–145.

Rapoport, L. (1965). The state of crisis: Some theoretical considerations. In H. J. Parad (Ed.), *Crisis intervention: Selected readings* (pp. 23–31). New York: Family Service Association of America.

Taplin, J. R. (1971). Crisis theory: Critique and reformulation. *Community Mental Health Journal, 7*(1), 13–23.

Selye, H. (1956). *The Stress of Life.* New York: McGraw-Hill.

SUGGESTED READINGS

Baldwin, B. A. (1980). "Styles of crisis intervention: Toward a convergent Model." *Journal of Professional Psychology, 11,* 113–20.

Burgess, A. W., & Baldwin, B. A. (1981). *Crisis intervention theory and practice: A clinical handbook.* Englewood Cliffs, New Jersey: Prentice-Hall.

Caplan, G. (1963). Emotional crisis. *Encyclopedia of Mental Health, 2,* 521–532.

Caplan, G. (1964). *Principles of preventive psychiatry.* New York: Basic Books.

Golan, N. (1969). When is a client in crisis? *Social Casework, 50*(7), 389–394.

Lindemann, E. (1965). Symptomatology and management of acute grief. In H. J. Parad (Ed.), *Crisis intervention: Selected readings.* (pp. 7–21). New York: Family Service Association of America. (Reprinted from *American Journal of Psychiatry,* 1944, *101*(2), 141–148)

Lindemann, E. (1956). The meaning of crisis in individual and family. *Teacher College Record, 57,* 310.

Parad, H. J. (1971). Crisis intervention. In *Encyclopedia of Social Work* (Vol. 1, pp. 196–202). New York: National Association of Social Workers.

Rapoport, L. (1965). The state of crisis: Some theoretical considerations. In H. J. Parad (Ed.), *Crisis intervention: Selected readings* (pp. 22–31). New York: Family Service Association of America.

2

Theoretical Knowledge Base for Crisis Intervention

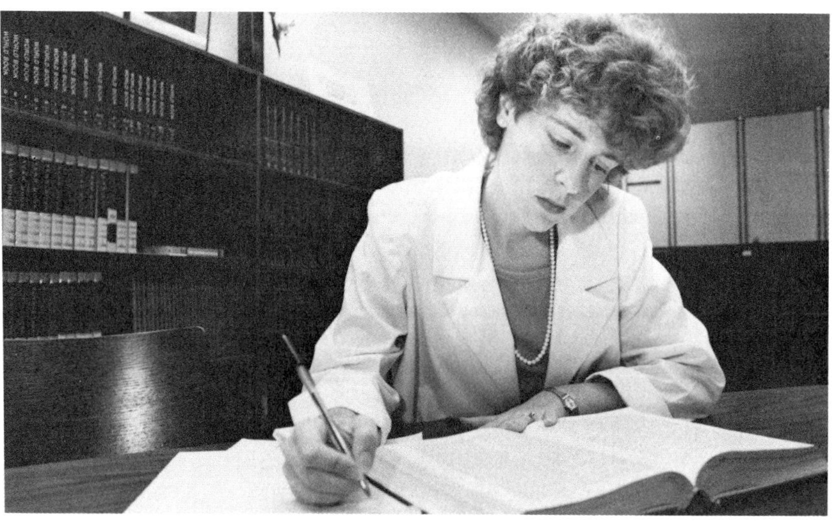

Case Studies

Doug, a 44-year-old man, requested an immediate appointment at the crisis center to discuss his concerns about things that had been happening to him. When he came in a few hours later, he stated that he had not been able to bounce back from failing his doctoral comprehensive examinations. Doug said that failing the exams, though not uncommon, was more important to him than to other students because of his age and responsibilities in life. He had switched from a field in which he had been quite successful to a totally new and unrelated field that required a doctorate. Now he was ashamed to tell his wife, who had returned to work after 15 years so he could pursue his goals, that he had flunked the test. He did not think that he could get his old position back because it had been more than two years since he had left it. Doug expressed intense feelings of self-depreciation and unworthiness. He felt that he had not only failed himself, but much worse, he had failed his wife and family. He did not know what he was going to do and felt like taking his life. Having come from a religious family, he recognized that the thought of taking his own life meant that he was at the final point of despair, and so he sought help immediately.

A middle-aged woman named Rosemary called the crisis center for an immediate appointment. She was in a state of panic because she had found a note from her husband Frank in which he spoke of suicide. Her husband was in love with another woman, whom he said he wanted to marry, but Rosemary had refused to give him a divorce. Rosemary and Frank had been married for 21 years, and she felt that his affair with the young woman was a passing fancy. He had been a loyal husband and a good father for all those years. On that basis she felt that he was having some "mental problems" and that he would snap out of it. However, since the affair had been going on for several months, the night before she found the note Rosemary had informed Frank that she was going to tell his mother about his behavior.

From our understanding of the concept of crisis, we can see that both Doug and Rosemary were in crisis. Their feelings of helplessness, overwhelming emotionality, and diminished cognitive functioning were typical, so they turned to someone else for help. In the first case, the crisis was resolved; Doug regained cognitive control of himself so that he was able to work out a plan with his professors to take the comprehensive examinations a second time. In the second case, Frank eventually committed suicide. Why were Doug and Rosemary (and Frank) in crisis? What caused their specific reactions to their precipitating events when others face the same kinds of problems with much less trouble? Why did they behave the way they did? We can find the answers in basic human behavior patterns. This chapter provides a basis for understanding human behavior that will help the therapist assess and evaluate the clients' social functioning and guide the therapeutic intervention.

While crisis theory does not require specific adherence to any one of the traditional theories of human behavior, a systematic theoretical approach to understanding social functioning is essential for maximum effectiveness and success. Intervention that is not based on some theory is a trial-and-error process; it leaves success too much to chance. A basic knowledge of theory gives the therapist greater control over the intervention situation. Some intellectual control is needed to reduce the unwanted emotional involvement that working with people in crisis entails. Some cognitive control helps the therapist develop confidence in his or her professional skills and abilities, which in turn helps the client (Goldstein, 1962). The therapist who feels confident is likely to project an image of strength and ability to deal with difficult problems.

Perhaps most important, theory allows the therapist to make predictions and thus to assess and evaluate the client's condition as a road map for intervention.

UNDERSTANDING HUMAN BEHAVIOR

There are many ways to conceptualize human behavior. Although each person who experiences a crisis is a unique individual, a broad perspective and relatively comprehensive study of human behavior is more useful in the long run than a single-subject study. Regardless of their individuality, all people in crisis have certain common characteristics. The therapist needs a comprehensive understanding of human behavior from which to begin.

We can start with some basic assumptions about human behavior:

1. All human behavior has a cause, and the causes always involve many complex interpersonal interactions between the individual and other people and the environment.
2. Human behavior is purposeful. People try to satisfy needs, to adapt to the social environment, and to defend against any stimulus that threatens their emotional equilibrium.
3. All human beings experience the same feelings and behaviors. The basic differences between people are not differences of kind but of degree.
4. The individual and his or her social environment are a united, interactional field.
5. Stress and conflict are an inevitable part of life. To live happily and productively, human beings must learn patterns of behavior that let them maintain and restore a sense of equilibrium.
6. The way a person functions psychosocially is the accumulative result of his or her life experiences and socialization process.
7. Effective social functioning is related to the nature of biological endowment, the social environment, and specific phases of the life cycle.
8. An individual's social functioning can range from highly effective to ineffective.
9. Psychosocial dysfunction can be ameliorated by assessing and evaluating contributing factors in the individual and the environment, and by intervening therapeutically.

Since we are concerned with a relatively comprehensive perspective of human behavior, let us begin with the human being's beginning, with biological behavior and its contribution to psychic development and social functioning.

Biological Determinants of Human Behavior

Although the human infant is born helpless, most are also born with specific capacities that will eventually enable them to function independently and ensure their own survival over time. Two factors affect that outcome: heredity and environment, the sum of experiences. While the individual's heredity is determined by the time of birth, the environment is not. The rest of this chapter explores how biological, psychological, and social experiences result in a specific psychic system and habitual patterns of social functioning.

The Family: Socialization and Personality Development

The family is a human group that is different than any other group. It lasts longer, offers more intense feelings, and provides more functions for the individual. It is the group most responsible for psychological development, emotional interaction, self-esteem, and identity. An individual's specific needs, values, and goals are first established in the family and later pursued and elaborated upon in adulthood. For most human beings the family is the most prolific contributor to the individual's psychic system. Thus, the subjective aspects of a crisis can often be understood through family background and experiences.

Human babies are born with the capacity to communicate their needs to their primary caretakers and to adapt to the social environment. These capacities allow the otherwise helpless infant to survive. Although the infant's basic potentials are innate, the way they develop is determined by the individual's specific social experiences. If the baby is to learn, the baby must be stimulated and have social experiences conducive to that end. In contrast to other animals, human beings can use their experiences not only to survive and adapt, but also as creative tools.

The human infant is also born with a need for affection. This need for nurture, coupled with the biological drive for survival, leads to interaction between the baby and the caretaker. This interaction is the infant's first social experience.

The next social experiences most infants have are within the family. The family is a system of interacting personalities, the basic purpose of which is the satisfaction of the needs of its members within the parameter of a specific social situation. The family is the agency that begins the socialization process. No adequate replacement has been found for the family in molding the child's personality and preparing the child for independent social functioning. Specifically, family experiences determine the way the infant thinks and learns, the infant's way of loving and being loved, self-concept and identity, and feelings of self-worth, security, self-confidence, responsibility, and trust. Let us look a little closer at this process.

Even before birth, the human child lives in a psychosocial climate affected by the personalities of the parents. The parents' own childhoods and life experiences determine how they relate to their children. Their feelings about pregnancy, the quality and nature of their marriage, and the mother's physical and emotional health during pregnancy all determine the kind of environment the infant is born into.

Birth interrupts the comfort of the fetal state and thrusts the child into a new world that brings pain and discomfort. The infant's level of activity after birth varies from one case to another. Some infants are more sensitive and less tolerant of aversive stimuli; others are more cuddly and responsive. The baby's biological behavior evokes responses in the parents, who give this behavior a personal interpretation and meaning. This interaction is the beginning of the cumulative social interaction between parent and child. Again it is the parents who give the infant's biological behavior its psychosocial meaning. This meaning influences the way the parents relate to the child; some parents interpret it as the child's feelings for them. For example, one father said, "I knew my child did not love me from the beginning because he stiffened up everytime I picked him up." At this point the infant's behavior was purely a biological reflex, perhaps in response to the feeling of being moved. But the father's personality and feelings led him to interpret the child's behavior and *respond to his own interpretation.* This in turn, if repeated often, could communicate negative feelings to the infant (Pemberton and Benady, (1973)).

At this point in the infant's life, the most important thing is the absence of pain; that is, the infant needs sleep, nourishment, and pleasurable sensations such as stroking. Research has shown that the infant's need for stroking and tactile stimulation beyond tension reduction is as vitally important for adequate psychosocial development as food is to the body. Bullard, Glaswer, Heagarty, and Pivchech (1973), Ribble (1944), and Spitz (1945) found that some children's will to live was greatly affected by the lack of interpersonal and affectional experiences. When the infant experiences pain, the reaction is automatic; the infant cries and contorts face and body as if its life were in danger. This reaction is purely in the service of survival; it is so urgent because the infant's psychic system is not developed enough to let him identify the source of the pain. This confusion is the prototype of the feelings of anxiety. The same phenomenon occurs in adults in anxiety. While experiencing anxiety, adults react with physiological responses as if their lives were in danger. More will be said about this under the topic of anxiety.

As time passes, the infant internalizes experiences and learns that the parents or caretakers are the source of feeding and pleasure and provide for the elimination of pain and discomfort. This recognition activates a bond of love that will have infinite influence on the child's psychic development throughout life (Bowlby, 1969, Lamb, 1977). It is one of the major considerations in understanding depression, as we shall see later. After needs have been satisfied repeatedly, the child develops confidence that they will be satisfied. The child soon learns that crying brings a parent, giving purpose to his or her behavior. Mental functioning starts when the child can recognize a purpose for behavior, perhaps when he or she stops crying at the sight of parents, before needs have been satisfied.

As the infant develops the certainty that biological needs will be satisfied in an environment of love and security, attention and learning can be directed toward higher psychosocially determined needs and adaptation to the social environment. If, on the other hand, the satisfaction of biological needs is threatened or inadequate, the basis for adequate social functioning is proportionately reduced and behavior continues to be biologically motivated.

As biological needs are satisfied and recede into the background on the basis of confidence created by repeated satisfaction, psychosocially determined needs assume the same urgency that biological needs once did. Now the need for love, affection, achievement, and so on, can produce disequilibrium. Now the stimulus for behavior is not just the satisfaction of biological needs but the satisfaction of psychosocial needs, a vital source of pleasure.

The process of psychic development is further complicated by the demands and prohibitions of the social environment (i.e., parents, social institutions, peers), which establishes not only what needs are valuable but also how they must or can be satisfied. Consequently the child must learn about his or her environment. At the same time, children must reconcile their own needs and desires with the nature of the environment in which they find themselves. Fortunately the human being has the potential to adapt to the environment. The way each individual adapts is determined by the specific nature of the social environment, beginning with the parents. They set the stage for love, values, goals, and the pursuit of happiness. Recall in the case of Rosemary and Frank that the event that led to Frank's suicide note was Rosemary's threat to tell his mother about his behavior. Not only is a child dependent on parents for survival, but the bond of love, or lack of it, established in infancy affects the individual throughout life. When the child reaches adulthood, love for another adult becomes as instrumental in psychic functioning as parental love once was.

In effect, human love represents a lifelong continuum. There are four important characteristics of human love. First, it is individually and idiosyncratically defined. Consider the battered wife who says she stays with her husband who beats her because she loves him. Second, the basis for love is an individual's feelings of self-worth and value. Third, many human activities (e.g., work, creativity) can be substitutes for love, either enhancing it or destroying it. Consider the husband who claims that he works 14 hours each day because he loves his family. This is fine if the family also perceives it as love. Fourth, love is not given unconditionally. As the child grows, this is learned quickly. The child must do certain things or refrain from doing certain things to please his or her parents. These demands do no harm if the parents love the child, if they are consistent in their responses, and clear and unambiguous in their expectations or communication. If the parents are happy with each other and their lives, if they understand, then it is not difficult for a child to please parents. However, family emotional and interactional relationships are complicated. In sum, love is individually and subjectively defined; this is why it is so difficult to describe what love is generally. Perhaps the most useful measure is the definition given by Freida Fromm-Reichman (1950). She says that mature love is being as concerned about the welfare of the loved one as you are about your own. Now let us discuss further parental influence on personality development.

Parents are two different individuals who enter a relationship with distinct pasts that affect their motivation for selecting each other. These motivations may or may not be compatible with each other. In addition, parents bring to their relationship their own individual personalities, including their ideas of motherhood and fatherhood. The roles of mother and father are greatly influenced by their relationship and their experiences with their own parents.

As children mature they begin to manifest their own will, and function independently. At this time the socialization process really begins, particularly if the child is restricted and prohibited from satisfying curiosity and meeting needs immediately and expediently. At some point the child's will clashes with the social environment (i.e., parents). The child's first conflict situation is whether to please self or to please parents. It does not matter to the child that the parents are acting in his own best interest. The child is driven by the desire for pleasure, which is influenced and limited by the threat of losing parental love or suffering some form of punishment if a behavior is unacceptable to them. At this point the child has several options: (a) attempt to satisfy needs impulsively and expediently, thereby risking rejection and punishment by parents; (b) abandon the need or desire and pretend that the need did not exist or was not wanted in the first place; (c) find a substitute satisfaction or disguise the original need; (d) satisfy this need in a manner that is pleasing to the parents, thereby retaining their affection and avoiding their punishment and disapproval. Much of psychic development involves reconciling internal needs with external opportunities, demands, limitations, and prohibitions. How children learn to resolve these conflicts to satisfy needs, values, and goals is part of the socialization process. Through this process the child evolves a specific psychic system.

PSYCHIC SYSTEM

The psychic system is a dynamic organization of mental faculties, the accumulation of all the individual's life experiences, psychic as well as social, from birth to its completion near the end of adolescence (although many theorists believe that this system is completed by age six). It is responsible for the individual's social functioning and specific ways of thinking, perceiving, feeling, and behaving. It is responsible for the individual's sensitivities. It ensures one's survival within the environment. Perception, memory, intelligence, language, and mobility are capacities of the psychic system. As a consequence of internalizing parental standards, values, and expectations, the child develops a conscience that helps regulate behavior according to past experiences. The child also seeks pleasure. All of these are forces in the personality, and their purpose is to make the individual a fully functioning self-actualizing person. However, to achieve these purposes, such forces must be coordinated and regulated. The ego, or self-system, or the individual's learned patterned responses, has this unifying purpose. Through the years of socialization and learning, one learns to maintain equilibrium while satisfying needs, pursuing goals, and meeting the demands of the social environment. However, one generally has little control over outside events. Thus each individual develops habitual patterns or methods of coping with conflicting demands and unusually significant upsetting events while remaining organized. These patterns are carried out routinely until some event overtakes the psychic system and attacks it at a vulnerable time.

Two important factors that stimulate psychic functioning and human behavior are self-concept and needs. It is the satisfaction of these two impelling factors that determines psychic equilibrium and the adequacy of social functioning. When either is threatened, some degree of disequilibrium results. We saw this in the cases presented at the beginning of the chapter. Doug's self-concept was threatened by his failure; Rosemary's needs for love and security were threatened by Frank's affair with a younger woman. To understand better, let us look at these two psychic forces in more depth.

Self-concept

Self-concept is how individuals see themselves. It is who each individual believes himself or herself to be, identity, the sum of what one stands for, one's beliefs, occupation, roles assumed, and on and on.

The self-concept is a fluid, changing gestalt, a referent for a person's activities. At any moment it gives a person either a sense of self, "I feel like I can be my real self," or the lack of it, "I feel I am not being myself now" or "I am afraid to be my real self here." It is the value judgment that we place on ourselves, mainly as a result of early perceptions of parental feelings and the tremendous human need to be loved and accepted, first by parents and later by significant others. Of course, the child's perception of the parents feelings about him or her may not be what the parents really feel; however, what is important is the *perception*, the individual's psychic reality. During early development the child internalizes parents' feelings, behavioral expectations, and demands into his or her own psychic system. The parents evaluate the child's behavior as good or bad, acceptable or unacceptable. Most children cannot separate their actions from their selves. They feel that who they are is determined by what they do. When they do something "good" that pleases their parents, they feel good about themselves. When the child does something unacceptable, the action is translated into, "I am no good" or "I am bad." The child internalizes external experiences as part of self-concept. A very important part of maturity is the separation of the internalized parental perception of what and who the individual is and the establishment of one's own self-concept and identity. This separation is not easy to accomplish because parents have such an early and lasting influence on psychic development. Consider the following example of parental influence on self-concept and behavior.

Anne, a 27-year-old married mother of three children, complained that she no longer felt worthwhile or of value just being a housewife; she said she wanted to get a job. She expressed these feelings to her mother, who made her feel guilty about them because her children still needed her. Anne's husband was in favor of and supported her desire to get a job. Ann revealed her conflict when she said, "I could never please my mother." As a part of Anne's socialization process, she had internalized her mother's values of motherhood. This would have been all right had they been Anne's values also. However, as Anne's feelings about being a housewife changed, she also wanted to change her self-concept and feelings about herself. At age 27, still needing her mother's approval, she felt considerable tension between pleasing her mother and pleasing herself. She felt that if she took a job, she risked losing the love and acceptance of her mother. The conflict would probably have occurred even if her mother had not directly interfered, because her mother's values and perception of her had been internalized. For Anne to resolve this conflict, she needed help in overcoming the feelings of the internalized mother.

While there are other explanations for the origin of self-concept, it is clearly an important variable in human behavior, one no therapist can afford to ignore. It originates in the process of identification in which children want to be like parents. This process facilitates adaptation to society and ensures its continuity. A good or at least adequate self-concept generally means satisfactory social functioning. When self-concept is poor, though, social functioning is ineffective. A threat or attack on an individual's self-concept can precipitate a crisis, as we saw in Doug's failing his doctoral comprehensive examinations.

Human Needs

Needs are also impelling forces that initiate and maintain human behavior. Specifically, a need is an internal stimulus experienced as tension that can be reduced by a specific source of satisfaction. The stronger the need, the greater the tension. The need-satisfaction sequence is as follows:

Need	→	**Action**	→	**Process**	→	**Satisfaction**
Stimulus and tension		*Behavior*		*Methods used to satisfy need*		*Tension reduction*

The satisfaction of a need is pleasurable. But neither the individual nor society is so constituted that all human needs can be satisfied unequivocally. Consequently, needs can be ranked in a hierarchy of relative potency. When one need is satisfied, another appears.

Hence human behavior is the satisfaction of one need after another. Some of the most powerful needs are for survival, sex, aggression, love, acceptance, self-esteem, recognition, achievement, value, and security. Human behavior can be understood in terms of need disposition. Not only can common stimuli such as longings for love or security serve as needs, uncommon stimulation can also be needed. For example, the need for punishment, the need for excitement, or the need to face danger can all lead certain people to act (e.g. mountain climbing, sky diving).

As long as needs are being satisfied, the individual can function adequately. If needs cannot be satisfied, frustration and social dysfunctioning can result. The degree of debilitation depends on the strength of the need, its significance for the maintenance of adequate social functioning, the methods used to satisfy the need, and the availability of sources of alternate satisfaction. The length of time that one can tolerate disequilibrium resulting from unsatisfied needs without breaking down is one's frustration tolerance.

Each society not only sets forth which needs are acceptable, but also establishes certain limits on the ways these can be satisfied. Thus each individual must reconcile the existence and the satisfaction of needs with the structure of the social environment. This makes intrapsychic conflict, that is, conflict within the psyche, inevitable. In such cases a person has four alternatives: (a) to satisfy the need directly and suffer the consequence; (b) to submit to the will of the opposing force and pretend that the need never existed; (c) to reduce the tension of the need by fantasy and wish fulfillment; or (d) to develop some compromise need as a substitute. The mind must develop ways to deal with powerful needs that cannot be directly satisfied. After discussing the concepts of identity and motivation, we will discuss several methods of adaptation to conflict.

IDENTITY

Identity has been given a great deal of attention in adolescence but comparatively neglected in adulthood. However, researchers have found that identity is a very important factor to the psychosocial functioning of adults. Therefore, we may conclude that it is also important in the development of a crisis condition, Identity is the integrative effect of feelings, needs, and roles that give a person a sense of individuality, worth, and purpose that is recognized by oneself and others (Dixon and Sands, 1983). When an event occurs that is perceived by an individual to be a threat to his or her identity (that is, an event defined as threatening a variety of one's roles and activities) and usual coping methods are ineffective, the individual experiences feelings of identity loss or diffusion; specifically, feelings of worthlessness, loss of purpose, and meaning. When one loses identity as symbolized by love, relationship, work, and social roles, the individual experiences a crisis.

MOTIVATION

Understanding motivation is important to understanding human behavior. Motivation is the desire to satisfy a need or to achieve a goal. It is both the reason for certain behavior and the force that impels a person to action.

The significance of motivation in our understanding of human behavior stems from the following premise:

a. The individual knows what he or she needs at the present or wants to accomplish.
b. The individual has methods that alert him or her to whether learned ways will be successful in the current situation.
c. Based on perception, the individual will attempt either to meet needs and achieve goals by past learned methods or devise new ones.
d. There are acceptable ways to satisfy needs and to achieve goals psychologically, interpersonally, and socially.
e. In general, people are sensitive to rejection as well as to failure to satisfy need and goals. Consequently, a great deal of the motivation for satisfying needs is to avoid failure just as much as it is to achieve goals.

For these reasons, motivation and behavior are not always open, honest, and forthright. They are often fraught with deceit, camouflage, and deviousness.

All human behavior, regardless of significance, is motivated and purposeful. Because needs are experienced as tension, the reduction of tension is motivation for the satisfaction of needs. This sounds simple, and it would be if people and societies were so constituted that all needs could be unequivocally satisfied. But such is not the case.

Motivation can exist on three levels: the conscious level, the preconscious level, and the unconscious level. One is aware of *conscious* motivation. For example, a crisis therapist might say that she wants to work with people in crisis in order to "help people." It follows therefore that for that therapist helping people satisfies a specific need. The therapist will continue to help people as long as the need exists and can be satisfied in that manner. Conscious motivation is generally realistic and truthful and should be accepted when the rational part of the psychic system is functioning without interference.

The *preconscious* level of motivation is that explanation or purpose that a person may have forgotten but that can be recalled fairly easily with some stimulation. The degree of preconscious motivation may vary, but for the most part it is generally close to that which is socially and personally acceptable. To use our crisis therapist as an example of preconscious motivation, she might recall that another reason for wanting to work with people in crisis was that it was the only job available at the time. Preconscious motivation is generally harmless and the product of forgetting and consciousness priorities.

Unconscious motivation is behavior that one is unaware of and cannot offer any rational explanation for when made aware of it. Unconsciously motivated behavior may be either constructive or destructive, but it is generally detrimental. When it is constructive, it is constructive in outcome only, since its success is so reinforcing that there is generally no need to question why one acts. Unconscious motivation is detrimental when its consequences are destructive. For example, if the crisis therapist works so hard at helping people that her family is neglected, some question of unconscious motivation could be raised.

While unconscious motivation is important, one should not become preoccupied with hidden meanings. Simply remember that people do, say, or think many things without logical explanations. They appear at times to be motivated by unknown forces. This is especially true of the person in crisis. Nevertheless, whatever he or she does has some basis, some purpose, some meaning. In such cases it is often necessary for the person to discover his or her own motivation as part of the cognitive restoration process. Because all motivation has to be described by the individual or inferred by any outsider, the therapist must be aware of the influence of motivation in the causes of human behavior. For instance:

Case Study

Ben called an agency in a state of crisis precipitated by his wife's leaving him. During the interview he revealed that his wife left him after he beat her because she did not want to become pregnant. He had beaten her before; each time she left, only to return the same day. This time she did not return, and Ben developed a state of panic. He rationalized away his beating of his wife as evidence of how much he loved her and could not stand to live without her. However, after four sessions he could accept the fact that his motivation for beating his wife was not that he loved her so much but that he wanted her to leave him so that he could justifiably return home to live with his mother. Follow-up one year later revealed that he was doing well living with his mother and had no desire to contact his wife, whom he had not seen since her leaving precipitated the crisis.

Ben's story shows how unconscious motivation can influence human behavior. Since motivation can be disguised in numerous ways, making a person aware of his or her true motivation can be very helpful. It will enable the individual to be able to handle the problem directly with appropriate methods and without the need for subterfuge. A simple example is that of a lawyer who tells a client who consults him relative to a small case, "Your case would cost ten times more to litigate than it is worth. You cannot afford me." The lawyer's motivation is to imply "I'm too good and superior for you." The lawyer, of course is not aware of what he means. If he were made aware of his motivation, in the next case he should present the cost of litigation in a direct manner and let the client decide whether it is affordable.

NATURE OF HUMAN CONFLICT AND COMMON COPING MECHANISMS

The maladaptive management of an internal conflict precipitated by an external event can result in a crisis condition. Conflicts and their resolutions are parts of daily living. Learning to resolve conflicts as part of the socialization process results in the establishment of habitual patterns of adaptation necessary for adequate social functioning.

Conflict, by definition, is a clash between at least two opposing forces of equal stength. In essence, any obstruction to the satisfaction of a highly motivated need can produce conflict. Tension is the essence of true conflict. Recall that the ultimate goal of the human being is to maintain equilibrium. Tension, however, upsets equilibrium; it is painful. Consequently, whenever tension occurs, some means must be found to get rid of it, restoring the individual to relative constancy. As Menninger (1963) states, "All human behavior represents the endeavor on the part of an organism to maintain a relatively constant inner and outer environment by promptly correcting all upsetting eventualities." The sources of conflict are innumerable.

Reference has already been made to the inevitability of conflict in the socialization process and personality development. It first occurs when the child matures to the point that individual needs, desires, or will clashes with those of the parents. It also should be kept in mind that the psychic system can control and manage conflict and still satisfy most needs within the limits of the social environment. The psychic system can also succumb to conflict and give way to impulsiveness and primitive satisfaction of needs if the need is strong enough and the opposition to its satisfaction is weaker. Evidence of this is seen in adults who fall back into various primitive behaviors such as temper tantrums, uncontrolled anger, fighting, and even murder to satisfy needs as a reaction to frustration or to release tension caused by unmet needs, deprivation, or threat to psychic values.

Intrapsychic conflict results from the discrepancy between internalized social standards and the desire to violate them or function differently. Conflict can arise when there is a desire to defy or deviate from one's upbringing. For example, intrapsychic conflict can result from the Catholic Church's position on abortion versus the sociolegal position. It occurs also when it is felt that one has failed to meet personal standards. It can occur when there is a desire to satisfy forbidden needs and strong counterforces prevent such satisfaction. Consider Brian, a college student who grew up in a strict environment in which he developed a strong conscience that prohibited drinking alcohol or the kind of partying that is typical of university students. He is now confronted with the quandary of whether to violate his upbringing, thereby feeling that he will lose the love and respect of his parents while gaining the acceptance of his peers, or lose the support of his peers while retaining good feelings about his behavior. Again, for this to be true intrapsychic conflict, both goals must be equally desirable, and a decision either way results in dire consequences. Intrapsychic conflict always involves incompatible forces competing for satisfaction.

Another source of intrapsychic conflict is the human being's capacity to symbolize, to let objects and experiences come to represent other real objects or experiences that at one time were significant. For example, hearing a song that you associate with a particular person can bring to mind images and feelings you had about that person. Because a symbol is only representative of the actual experience or object and is not the real experience or object, there is always some degree of emotional distortion or exaggeration. The symbolized experience can never be reexperienced as it actually happened but only as it is remembered. The majority of intrapsychic conflicts significant to crisis therapy involve opposition between significantly powerful needs that are in conflict with one's conscience and interpersonal relationships. Such situations are illustrated by conflict over sexual mores, religion, or the desire to express undesirable behavior or satisfy personally unacceptable feelings or needs. Conflict always involves incompatible forces competing for satisfaction. Conflict per se is not bad, since successful resolution contributes to learning and growth. In fact, Erikson (1963) bases his theory of psychosocial development on a conflict model (e.g., trust versus mistrust, and so on).

The psychic system enables the individual to develop an array of coping mechanisms used to reduce or alleviate the tension resulting from either unresolved conflict or any other condition that makes it necessary for the individual to guard against threats to the integrity of the self. These coping mechanisms not only reduce tension, thus helping to maintain equilibrium, but they also aid adaptation. Everyone uses them to some extent. Hence a coping mechanism is any mental process or behavioral manifestation used to avoid or relieve painful affect and aid adaptation regardless of origin. Such mechanisms are also called *defense mechanisms, mental mechanisms,* or *dynamisms.* Coping mechanisms are prophylactic in nature; they do not resolve conflict or problems. Although they are used to some extent by everyone, they become detrimental when they are used exclusively, and prevent the individual from assuming responsibility for solving a problem or taking necessary action to change a situation when to do so is in the individual's best interest. Many of the coping mechanisms become a part of the individual's habitual patterns of adaptation and often facilitate problem-solving methods by preventing the psychic system from becoming overwhelmed with painful affect. Some people, for example, cope with depression by excessive sleeping. Others may cope by a special kind of physical exercise. Coping mechanisms are generally ineffective for the person in crisis for one or more of the following reasons: (a) they are used as a substitute for realistic problem-solving methods; (b) they are used to unduly falsify reality; (c) they are used excessively, preventing the individual from understanding and assuming responsibility for personal behavior; (d) they fail to prevent the individual from becoming overwhelmed with emotions. Part of the process of crisis evaluation is determining what habitual patterns of coping mechanisms the individual is using and why they are not effective. A discussion of some of the major and more generally accepted coping mechanisms used by people in crisis will further the understanding of human behavior.

Repression. Repression is the process by which unacceptable or unmanageable experiences, feelings, ideas, acts, or needs are automatically and without conscious awareness made unconscious because conscious awareness would result in painful, unacceptable, or deleterious consequences. Repressed feelings are not permanently lost or forgotten. They are pushed deep into the unconscious part of the mind. However, to keep them unconscious requires energy. Sometimes when events in daily life require additional energy, the amount of energy available for repression is reduced, and the repressed feelings, needs, or drives tend to manifest themselves either indirectly or directly. That which is repressed ranges from current situations to significant early childhood feelings and conflicts. Repression functions rather like forgetting, except that it occurs at a much deeper level and is much more significant to social functioning. According to Anna Freud (1966), "repression consists of the withholding or the expulsion of an idea or affect from the conscious ego."

In effect, repression is one way in which an individual can cope with conflict or any other source of pain that cannot be coped with consciously. That which is repressed is still laden with energy and presses for expression and satisfaction. An unresolved conflict may remain throughout each phase of personality development but may be kept from interfering with social functioning through the process of repression. But remember, that which is repressed strives for satisfaction, and keeping it repressed requires counterenergy of the ego. As long as the counterenergy is greater than the strength of the repression, equilibrium can be maintained.

However, ego energy needed to maintain repression is not always the same. Several functions can reduce ego energy used to maintain repression, specifically, using alcohol or drugs; sleep (during which repressions can be manifested in dreams); intense changes in physiological development or function, such as puberty; the withdrawing of various kinds of emotional needs, or deprivation; and as we have seen, events that threaten life or important values or needs. When repression fails, the significance of the old unresolved conflict forces the individual to ignore the current problem and to try once more to deal with the old conflict.

Dealing with pressure of the old conflict creates fewer feelings of helplessness and desperation than trying to deal with the current conflict or problems appearing to be insurmountable. This is supported by Rusk (1971, p. 250) when he talks about psychological regression:

> The overwhelmed ego, inadequate to manage the stimulus, manifests increasing anxiety with increasing regression to earlier (infantile) previously satisfying (pleasurable and/or anxiety reducing) behavior less in

touch with current reality, or more global ego, id, and superego regression to earlier but more manageable conflicts in which the anxiety level, although still present, is less overwhelming than in the current one.

It can be seen that whenever repression cannot be maintained, problems in psychosocial functioning can result. On the other hand, successful repression can aid and facilitate satisfactory social functioning and coping capacities.

Denial. Denial is a process by which an individual refuses to admit into conscious awareness some painful or unacceptable feeling or event that actually exists. Denial is similar to repression except that there is some implication of awareness in the necessity to deny. Denial operates more at a preconscious level than does repression. It can be used as a protection from a threatened loss of self-esteem and feelings of inadequacy or inferiority. A common example of the use of denial is the disbelief some people express when faced with the impending death of a loved one or close friend. A client may use denial when he says that his marriage is perfectly happy and he cannot understand why his wife wants to leave him. An elderly person may refuse to recognize deterioration of health by engaging in behavior that is detrimental.

Rationalization. Rationalization is the process by which excuses are used to make one's failures, disappointments, and painful feelings more acceptable. It can be used to justify behavior that would be harmful to self-esteem. It is used by everyone; everyone occasionally must account for personal defeats, misfortunes, or failures. Although rationalization is frequently offered after the fact, it can be used to reduce the pain of anticipated negative consequences.

Intellectualization. In this process, the individual turns unacceptable or painful feelings and needs into intellectual activities or discussions. The person may become preoccupied with some abstract subject such as philosophy, religion, or politics. Its primary purpose is to control painful feelings and emotions that would be intolerable otherwise. It is especially important for the crisis therapist to recognize, since it deprives the individual of needed emotional expression. Closely related to intellectualization is isolation. In that process, feelings normally associated with painful events are separated and pushed into the unconscious. In essence it is a repression of emotions normally accompanying a specific situation or event. Rather than controlling such feelings by talking abstractly, the individual who uses isolation behaves as if he or she has no feelings. It is easy to misconstrue isolated feelings because so frequently the lack of emotion is considered a sign of strength. For example, when a parent has gone through the traumatic loss of a child and remains in control, showing no sign of emotionality, many people interpret that behavior as a sign of strength. Isolation is detrimental when it prevents humanly required affective expression.

Displacement. Displacement is the process by which feelings are shifted from their original source to another source or object because of a perceived danger in directing them toward the true source. The perceived danger may or may not be real. Both positive and negative emotions can be displaced. The only requirement is the perception that to direct them where they belong is too dangerous. Scapegoating is an example of displacement. Another common example is the person who is angry at his boss but goes home and kicks his cat. The husband who has repressed hatred for his mother may be abusive to his wife as an unconscious substitute.

Reaction formation. This is the process by which manifest feelings and behavior are diametrically opposite to what is truly desired. Reaction formation is generally manifested by its excessive undesirable consequences. Maternal overprotection is an example. Another example is the wife who has repressed feelings of hate toward her husband and develops excessive concern for his welfare. Reaction formation can also take the opposite approach, in which behavior manifesting hate disguises strong feelings of love. The famous Johnny Cash song "A Boy Named Sue" illustrates this. Here the hard times given a boy named Sue makes him tough and he avoids any potentiality for being soft and unprepared for a hard life. Reaction formation to a fear of softness is excessive hardness or toughness.

Projection. In projection, individuals attribute their own painful, unacceptable feelings to someone else or to another situation to protect self-esteem or avoid feelings of weakness. The purpose of projection is to protect oneself from experiencing unacceptable or painful emotions. It prevents persons from assuming responsibility for their own behavior, and so long as it is used, change is difficult. It is the basis of suspiciousness and mistrust. A client who says the therapist dislikes him (assuming that is not true) may be hiding the feeling that he does not like the therapist.

Compensation. Compensation is the process by which the individual attempts to make up for some real or imagined shortcomings by some excessive activity designed for that purpose. Compensation is manifested by any exaggerated effort to attain distinction in any area of inadequacy or inferiority. Examples of compensation are numerous: the little person who acts aggressively, or the working parents who are oversolicitous toward the children because they feel guilty about neglecting them while finding satisfaction on the job. The need for compensation is subjectively determined, based on an absence of some value that is desirable.

Restitution. Closely related to compensation, restitution is the process by which a person amends and offers reparation to a person or group for wrongdoings, injuries, or damages for which he or she feels responsible. Restitution is used to alleviate guilt feelings and responsibility. For example, the father who feels guilty about punishing his child too severely may take her on a camping trip. Wrongdoings and guilt are the basis of the restitution mechanisms.

Identification. Identification is a very important mechanism in psychic development, used for ego reinforcement. It is the process by which individuals make characteristics of a loved or admired person an integral part of themselves. The attributes adopted may be feelings, behaviors, goals, ideas, or mannerisms. Identification is the process by which children learn to become like their parents. It is also the reason why famous persons are chosen to appear in commercials. Identification has great individual value because it makes persons feel better about themselves. It implies that identifying with the admired one will make him love you on the same basis that he loves himself, and you can love yourself for being like the admired one. However, in the case of parents and children it does not always work that way, since the child sometimes identifies also with the negative or rejected part of the parent. That is, there can be negative identification also. It should be emphasized, though, that identification is very important to self-love. It is also important in the helping relationship between the therapist and the client, and the therapist should be aware of it. It is necessary for the establishment of rapport and empathy.

Introjection. Introjection as used here is a special form of identification in which the perceived feelings of parents and significant others are internalized and experienced as part of the self. It is instrumental in the process of depression. We can see how it is manifested in the grieving process following the death of a loved one, in which the survivor feels and reacts as if a part of the self has been lost, or in the case of Anne, the mother of three who felt worthless as a housewife, in which introjection was a part of development of the self. The manifestation of introjection is less obvious than some of the other mechanisms. Consequently its usefulness here is the recognition that it results from the lengthy closeness with parents, whose relationship and experiences become introjected into the ego or psychic system.

Sublimation. Sublimation is the process by which unacceptable needs, desires, or impulses are directed into socially approved activities. Evidence of sublimation is generally the excessive zeal with which the individual is preoccupied with sublimated activity. It generally distracts the individual from being a well-rounded person. If the opportunity for sublimation fails, a crisis can develop. Athletics and professions such as medicine and law, requiring great amounts of education and training and advanced degrees, can be outlets for sublimated drives. When the outlet is blocked in some manner, a crisis may ensue.

Regression. Regression is a major mechanism exhibited by people in crisis. It is the process by which an individual returns to an earlier immature mode of feeling and behaving. Regression is illustrated by the child who has been toilet trained but begins to have frequent toilet accidents when the new baby is brought home. It is also illustrated by the middle-aged person who suddenly starts to act like an adolescent. We also see regression in the manifestations of anxiety and depression. Although regression generally occurs when one is unable to solve current problems, it can serve a constructive purpose. It is constructive during sleep and when it allows a person to return to a conflict situation stronger. It is deleterious when it is used as a permanent form of escape from problems in current reality.

Thus far the generally accepted coping mechanisms that relate most frequently to people in crisis have been discussed. Others will be discussed as they arise in special situations. It is important to recognize that coping mechanisms are means by which people maintain equilibrium. They become a part of their habitual patterns of adaptation. Consequently, being able to identify them and understand how they work and function is essential for understanding the crisis process. When the initial stress of the precipitating event is too great for the usual coping mechanisms, initial tension is experienced and social functioning begins to deteriorate. Progressively, then, to halt the process, the individual may move from his or her usual mode of rationalization to a more serious mechanism such as projection. If this mechanism restores equilibrium, the individual need go no further. If it does not, however, tension increases, requiring more elaborate measures. It is the failure of coping mechanisms that ultimately leads to a crisis state. How coping mechanisms function to maintain equilibrium and contribute to adaptation has been discussed. Attention can now be focused on what happens to the individual whose coping mechanisms and habitual patterns of adaptation are ineffective, leading to personality disorganization and a crisis state. The important question here is why an event causes a crisis in one person and not in another. We already know that it is not the event that causes the crisis, since the same event may be perceived as a healthy challenge to one person and not to another. It is the meaning of that event to the individual, the personal interpretation of danger to the individual. The emotional reaction to the perceived danger reduces the ability to cope with the problem. The more ineffective he or she is in dealing with the problem, the more emotional the individual becomes and the greater are the feelings of helplessness. Finally, the crisis state emerges.

If the danger of the event is subjectively determined, it is important to know what the precipitating event means to the person in crisis. Why is it personally interpreted as it is? The reason a person in crisis personally interprets the precipitating event as he or she does is revealed by the manifest reaction to the event. With the exception of suicide and homicide, almost all human reactions to events precipitating a crisis (i.e., catastrophes, illnesses, deaths, personal losses, values, and obstacles to happiness) are manifestations of anxiety or depression or their derivatives. Actually, even suicide and homicide are derivatives of anxiety and depression. Understanding the meaning, purpose, and function of these two universal emotions provides the key to understanding the person in crisis and the meaning to that person of the precipitating event. It also suggests the type of intervention needed.

ANXIETY

Anxiety is a powerful human emotion. It exists in everyone in varying degrees and under certain circumstances. The executive struggling with corporate decisions, the salesman failing to reach a quota, the adolescent rebelling against parents, and the student trying to balance classes, work, and family may all experience anxiety. Anxiety under such circumstances is so common that it can be called normal. However, the effect of anxiety on people can be both constructive or destructive, depending upon the intensity, duration, and cause. Its effect is constructive when there is just enough anxiety to generate energy and motivate people to solve problems and achieve. When anxiety exists beyond the optimal level, it can reduce effectiveness, causing mild confusion, or disorganization, or panic, depending upon the degree. In panic anxiety, the disintegration of the personality or psychic system is so great that destructive behavior to self or others can occur. Anxiety is central to a crisis. When it becomes so intense, so overwhelming that it is unmanageable, personality disorganization occurs and a crisis develops.

Although the coping mechanisms we have discussed have some adaptive value, basically they are used to avoid or alleviate anxiety. When they fail, anxiety develops. If relief is not forthcoming relatively soon, the threat of personality disorganization exists. This is why people so often become desperate to find a way to alleviate a crisis. If they do find a way, positive consequences result; if they do not, the best result that can be expected is some psychopathology or mental decompensation. As ineffective at resolving problems as most coping mechanisms are, they do reduce the effects of painful anxiety to a great degree. The debilitating effect of a crisis condition is determined by the degree of anxiety present.

But what is this powerful emotion? First, it is an innate physiological response to danger in the interest of survival. Its purpose is to prepare the human being for fight or flight by increasing the activity level of the body systems. As we saw, the prototype of anxiety is the infant's crying and contortions. The repeated experiences of being cared for, coupled with normal development and maturation, relegate much of the purely instinctual survival anxiety to the past. It is always there, however, and comes to the surface if life is threatened. The remainder serves as a psychological function. Any perceived danger to significant psychosocial needs can reactivate anxiety in the same way as when survival is at stake. Thus anxiety serves both survival and psychological purposes.

With this in mind, anxiety is defined as tension and apprehension resulting from the subjective anticipation of danger from an unknown source. To be useful as a psychological concept, anxiety should be distinguished from fear. It is easy to confuse the two, since the physiological reactions are the same for both. The cause distinguishes one from the other. Fear is the apprehension resulting from a known source that is inherently dangerous. The response is appropriate. In fear, the danger is real, objective, extrapsychic (e.g., a snake, a person with a gun). In anxiety the danger is subjectively determined; it is anticipated and unknown, internal and not readily determined. The source of anxiety is intrapsychic. Since the source of the danger is unknown, the individual has to engage in trial and error to try to escape from the danger, but what the individual seeks to escape from is the painful effect of the anxiety. However, as Schachtel (1959) states:

> The threat of anxiety as a potentiality can be eliminated only by the actual encounter with the dreaded situation or activity, because until we actually meet the situation we do not know whether and how we will be able to live with it, master it, or perish in it, and thus we cannot transform the unknown and new into something knowable and known. Such encounter means leaving the embeddedness in the familiar and going forth to an unknown meeting with the world.

It is for these reasons that people most often want to reduce and alleviate anxiety. However, anxiety is a universal human emotion, and it is "normal" for people to experience it. Most of the time the individual can find an excuse or justification for normal anxiety: a test, a new job, an important report due, a new situation. Furthermore, coping mechanisms usually are effective in controlling and reducing normal anxiety so that the person continues to function well. Normal anxiety is proportionately manageable and serves as a constructive motivating force for the individual to be responsible in order to prevent greater anxiety. For example, to prevent greater anxiety from the threat of failing a test, the student studies. When anxiety goes beyond normal limits, it renders the individual dysfunctional, and the goal becomes getting rid of the anxiety rather than having it serve as a constructive motivating force. When anxiety becomes overwhelming, it is diffuse and vague. The individual complains of a feeling of nervousness and worry and feels afraid of something but is not exactly sure what it is.

Manifestations of Anxiety

Overwhelming anxiety is a crisis state, and it is experienced and manifested in a variety of ways. The most common direct manifestations of anxiety are physiological and mental (psychomotor). Anxiety can affect almost every organ system in the human body. It makes a person feel as if there is something physically wrong. The most common physiological signs of anxiety are heart palpitation, flushing, tightness in the chest, inappropriate perspiration, increase in blood pressure, and rapid pulse. The individual may have tremors of various parts of the body such as the hands, or the entire body may shake. He or she may be restless or agitated, may pace the floor, or be unable to sit still. Sleep disturbances, insomnia, excessive sleeping, and disturbing dreams are common. There may be a persistent cough, or clogging of the throat or a dry mouth. There may be a complaint of stomach pains, cramps, or burning sensations. The stomach discomfort may be referred to as a "nervous stomach." The person's appetite is generally poor, or he or she may complain of difficulty keeping food in the stomach, nausea, diarrhea or frequent urination, headaches, and backaches. There may be reduced interest in sex or even some sexual dysfunctioning. A disturbance in the menstrual cycle is not unusual. Hives or other changes in the skin can be caused by anxiety.

Anxiety greatly reduces mental functioning. It is in this area that the crisis therapist must assess and evaluate in order to determine the client's capacity for continued social functioning and the kind of treatment indicated. Anxiety may be manifested in the individual's communication and speech patterns. There may be slurring of words, rapid speech, or loud talking. Logical thinking capacity may be impaired, as may judgment and decision making. Reality testing is most often affected. There may be poor or impaired concentration and attention span. There may be some confusion and poor memory. In essence, the emotionality affects normal mental capacity and leads to reduced social functioning.

Other indirect signs of anxiety include angry, hostile, or impulsive behavior. Various forms of acting out can be signs of anxiety; for example, behavior that is unusual for the individual such as sexual promiscuity, stealing, running away, excessive drinking, or drug use.

The Role of Anxiety for the Person in Crisis

Anxiety is one of the primary signs of a person in crisis. If an individual reacts to a precipitating event with anxiety, the basic meaning of the precipitating event to that individual is a perceived threat to survival, loss of impulse control (sex or aggression), bodily integrity, or some psychosocially determined need perceived to have a life or death value (e.g., "I cannot live without her"). Anxiety resulting from a threat to survival or bodily integrity can be easily understood (e.g., illness, catastrophe, and other real threats to life). Anxiety resulting from the threat to a psychosocial need requires more explanation. The basis of such anxiety is founded in the socialization process; specifically, in the human being's lengthy dependency on the mother or other caretaker for survival. When the child develops to the point that he or she can differentiate self from other objects and persons, the child recognizes that mother is the major source of the satisfaction of survival needs and feelings of love, protection, and security. Early interactions with parents are especially important to emotional development. As confidence and contentment are developed through parents' repeated satisfaction of needs, and as the human being progresses through life, the importance of such needs is transferred to significant others (spouse, friend, loved one), symbols (money, home), situations (job, position), goals, and values. Their loss or threatened loss can create anxiety, and the reaction is similar to a threat to survival. In reality the feeling being experienced is, "This loss or threatened loss is so important to my survival, to my living, that I do not feel that I can function without it." "It is so significant to my emotional integrity and well-being that I cannot function. I feel helpless and confused. I do not know what I am going to do." "Without it something dreadful is going to happen to me." "I am no longer protected." "I cannot go on." Anxiety creates a general feeling of helplessness, unprotectedness, abandonment, or fear of physical or bodily harm.

Clinical Anxiety

We have seen that anxiety is an important stimulus for human behavior. It is painful tension so disequalizing that adaptation and coping methods are developed to avoid, tolerate, or alleviate it. Despite its pain, anxiety seems to provide motivation for the process of growth and maturation as well as an impetus for maintaining psychic equilibrium (homeostasis). It requires inner resources to master it, thus aiding the capacity for self-control and delayed gratification. However, we have seen what happens to the person in crisis when anxiety becomes so intense that it cannot be handled.

This is a temporary state for those in crisis. For others, overwhelming anxiety exists for so long that maladaptation methods are developed. The purpose of these maladaptive methods, the patterns of which are called clinical syndromes, is to avoid and control anxiety. We call this clinical anxiety because it is the chronic result of intrapsychic conflict or a personality problem, contrasted to the individual in crisis who is reacting to the occurrence of a significant event which he or she cannot cope with by applying the usual coping methods. Anxiety exists in most of the clinical syndromes including schizophrenia. However, anxiety is central to a group of syndromes called anxiety disorders: anxiety states, phobia disorders, and obsessive-compulsive disorders. (Diagnostic and Statistical Manual-DSM-III, 1980).

In phobic disorders the anxiety is displaced onto an object or situation which externalizes the intrapsychic conflict. As long as the individual can avoid the phobic object, the anxiety can be controlled. If this is not possible, anxiety develops, often to a panic proportion depending upon the ability of the individual to get away from the phobic object. We can recognize a phobic disorder by the irrational and disproportionate reaction to the phobic object or situation. To repeat, phobias interfere with functioning when they cannot be avoided. In obsessive–compulsive disorders, the obsessive–compulsive behavior (thoughts, ruminations, rituals, and ceremonies) controls the anxiety associated with the intrapsychic conflict. In anxiety states the major disturbance is the experience of anxiety itself, which may be free-floating, or not attached to anything such as generalized anxiety disorders or panic disorders.

In the final analysis, clinical anxiety differs from normal anxiety only in cause and degree. It is the effect of the anxiety that is most significant.

Case Study

Keith, a 32 year old, has come to the mental health clinic complaining of a fear that he was going "insane." For several years, he had been feeling tense and nervous, with blurred vision and dizziness at times. For the past year, however, his nervous tension had gotten worse, making him irritable and unable to relax. He felt driven by excessive anxiety. Two days before coming to the clinic he had an anxiety attack and felt that he was dying. He managed to get to the hospital emergency room where the doctor found no organic cause for the symptoms and referred him to the clinic.

We can see from this summary that Keith had been attempting to cope with his problems for a long time, and his over-functioning had been affected by those efforts.

DEPRESSION

Depression, along with anxiety, is another major emotional manifestation of a crisis condition. Depression and anxiety represent opposite ends of the affective continuum. Anxiety results from the subjective anticipation of a perceived danger, manifested by disorganized hyperactivity and physiological changes in the interest of survival. It is basically a physiological response that facilitates the individual's preparation for fight or flight, but as we have seen, in crisis its excessiveness is debilitating. Clearly, anxiety—though disorganized and excessive—is the individual's effort to solve a problem even though he or she does not know how to do so.

In contrast, the opposite reaction occurs in depression. As Bibring (1953) states, "In extreme situations the wish to live is replaced by the wish to die." He continues to state:

> The feelings of helplessness are not the only characteristic of depression. On further analysis of the quoted and other instances one invariably finds the condition that certain narcissistically significant, i.e., for the self-esteem pertinent, goals and objects are strongly maintained. Irrespective of their unconcious implications, one may roughly distinguish between three groups of such persisting aspirations of the person: (1) the wish to be worthy, to be loved, to be appreciated, not to be inferior or unworthy; (2) the wish to be strong, superior, great, secure, not to be weak and insecure; and (3) the wish to be good, to be loving, not to be aggressive, hateful and destructive. It is exactly from the tension between these highly charged narcissistic aspirations on the one hand, and the ego's acute awareness of its (real and imaginary) helplessness and incapacity to live up to them on the other hand, that depression results.*

Depression is a *mood* disturbance characterized by feelings of sadness, inferiority, inadequacy, hopelessness, pessimism, dejection, self-depreciation, guilt or shame. The depressed individual may suffer from either insomnia or excessive sleeping. Most important, the individual looks and acts depressed. He or she may cry as though feeling helpless. Depending upon the degree, the depressed person's social functioning decreases as the abilities to think and concentrate are affected. The

*From "The Mechanisms of Depression" by E. Bibring, (1953), in *Affective Disorders: Psychoanalytic Contributions to Their Study*, P. Greenacre, (Ed.). New York: International University Press. Copyright 1953 by International University Press. Reprinted by permission.

depressed person may repeatedly complain about physical problems or lose interest in social relationships, work, and sex.

Normal Depression

Depression as a mood disturbance is not in itself psychopathological. Depression, like anxiety, is a universally experienced emotion. Everyone becomes depressed at one time or another. It may be called "feeling blue" or "feeling down" or "in the dumps." The executive experiencing anxiety about the prospects of making the right decision then becomes depressed if she makes the wrong decision. The salesperson becomes depressed when his bonus check fails to meet expectations because he did not reach his quota. Mild periods of depression occur more or less spontaneously, generally in association with events that affect our mood at the time. It may be a temporary setback, disappointment, or even the weather. The "down period," however, usually does not last longer than several days and does not unduly interfere with the individual's psychosocial functioning and responsibilities. Generally, a reasonable explanation based on the occurrence of an external event can be offered for the depressed state. A typical example of normal depression is the transient state of despondency and lethargy following a disappointment. It could be receiving a grade lower than expected, an unsatisfactory evaluation, a move to a new city either by oneself or a friend, or anything that affects self-esteem or some significant value or need.

Another normal depressive reaction is grief and bereavement, a form of depression caused by the death of a loved one. After a death it is normal to experience a grief reaction which can last indefinitely but generally from two months to a year. Bornstein, Clayton, Halikas, Maurice, and Robins (1973) found that only 17 percent of the grief reactors in their sample suffered from depression a year after the death of a loved one. It is not unusual for some depression to reoccur annually on the anniversary date of the death of the loved one. Although the depression may be intense and prolonged, the individual is able to function relatively effectively. The burden of painful feelings and emotions can be set aside as necessary in order to fulfill obligations and responsibilities. Although there may be a reduction in outside interests, there is some awareness of and responsibility to one's social network.

In normal depression the degree of guilt and loss of self-esteem is minimal. The individual is not a threat to himself or herself. Normal depression has basically the same symptoms as clinical depression; the difference, however, is in the intensity, duration, cause, and hopefulness. Above all, in normal depression, the individual is not depressed very long, is able to function effectively, and can offer a reasonable explanation for the cause of the depression and regain hope of improvement relatively quickly.

Depression In Crisis

Depression in a crisis state is a mood disturbance in which feelings of dejection, sadness, and despair are debilitating. Almost always, varying degrees of feelings of self-depreciation and unworthiness are expressed. The depressed person looks depressed and unhappy. Facial expression and posture reflect dejection and despair. The individual is generally pessimistic, feels helpless and very often hopeless. Sometimes suicidal intentions are present. There is generally a loss of interest in others, a tendency toward withdrawal, and preoccupation with self. Psychomotor retardation is manifested by lack of spontaneity and deliberate speech. Cognitive functioning and concentration are generally impaired. There are often physical complaints such as headaches or backaches. Constipation or gastrointestinal tract symptoms are often present; loss of appetite and insomnia are common. Guilt and self-blame are almost always involved, either directly or indirectly. There may be a preoccupation with thoughts of death or a wish to be dead. Sexual interest and affectionate feelings may decline. There may also be an excessive use of alcohol or drugs.

Origin of Depression

There are many explanations for the origin of depression. Freud said that it was similar to grief. The behavioral theorist says it is learned helplessness and loss of social reinforcement. The sociologist says that it results from loss of role status, and the existentialist says that it is the loss of meaningful existence. From this vantage point the basis of depression is twofold: (a) threats to the seemingly innate need for human relatedness, affection, and psychosocially determined values to sustain psychic equilibrium; and (b) the nature and qualitative development of self-concept, self-esteem, and self-worth.

Earlier, reference was made to coping mechanisms, including the internalization process, identification, or modeling. It is through these processes that the individual develops self-concept and self-values. Through socialization, a set of functional self-values operates at all times to influence social functioning. When events occur that threaten self-concept or self-values, they are experienced as a personal loss to self, causing depression. When this happens, developmental feelings about the self, including those believed to be of the parents, are reactivated. Hence the individual evaluates self according to his parents or her interpretation of the meaning of the event causing the depression. For example, when Doug failed his doctoral comprehensive examinations he equated the external event with his worth. In effect he said, "Since I failed the examinations, I am personally no good, worthless." Such evaluations are the result of previous demands, standards, expectations, and evaluations by others, especially parents. They are internalized and introjected into the individual psychic system, and functionally, individuals respond to themselves in ways similar to the way their parents did or their perception of what would be the parents' response to their behavior, performance, or achievements. In sum, at the same time that it is believed that, either directly or indirectly, another human being is invariably involved in causing depression, still another can help that individual through it. In other words, object relationships are both the cause and cure for depression. Depression is discussed further in chapter 6.

Precipitating Factors

Depression can overcome a variety of individuals and be precipitated by seemingly trivial, complicated, or serious events: the woman who became deeply depressed because she accidently broke her artificial fingernail; the wife who became depressed because she had to drive her husband's Cadillac instead of her own smaller car; the husband who became depressed because a flood destroyed his home for which he worked so hard; the wife who became deeply depressed because her husband of 20 totally unhappy and incompatible years of marriage divorced her.

Depression, regardless of the precipitant, has several salient characteristics. The individual experiences (a) a loss—a loved one, a valued possession, self-esteem, status, position, role, psychosocial need, or emotional support; (b) dominant feelings of being unloved and lonely; (c) feelings of helplessness, inadequacy, and inferiority; (d) a feeling of failure to meet other-determined internalized developmental standards. This singly means that the failure to meet internalized expectations of others is too important and has more than one meaning for the individual, usually with antecedent ties to parents or significant others from the past.

In sum, the causes of depression fall into two basic categories. The first is the loss or threatened loss of a love object or emotional support, self-esteem, status, position (e.g., economic failure), or role, and other ego values needed for psychic equilibrium. Feelings of being unloved and loneliness are the dominant features. The second cause of depression is failure to meet internalized standards, values, or goals. This category also includes violation of—or a wish to violate—moral values, right and wrong, good and bad, or the failure to achieve at a specific level. We saw such conditions in the cases of Rosemary and Doug.

Clinical Depression

Case Studies

Judy, a 27-year-old graduate student in chemistry, was brought to the mental health clinic by her roommate in a very depressed state. For more than two years, Judy had complained of unhappiness, feelings of inadequacy, low self-esteem, chronic fatigue, and a generally pessimistic outlook on life. Her roommate thought that her complaints were associated with her studies, with her role as a student, since her academic performance was passing but unsatisfactory according to her standards. During the prodromal period preceding the appointment at the clinic, Judy was able to muster feelings of well-being lasting from several days to a few weeks. About two months before the appointment at the clinic, Judy became increasingly depressed, and developed sleeping disturbances and inability to concentrate. Her appetite was very poor, and she steadily lost weight. This deepening of her depression occurred several days after a rejection she received from the medical-student husband of a friend of hers.

Isaac, age 40, was referred to the psychiatrist by the crisis therapist because of his severe depression. While Isaac was home, he spent most of his time sitting in a chair moaning and wringing his hands. He appeared severely dejected, and his eyes were red from weeping. His posture sagged when he periodically paced the floor. He refused to eat and ignored his personal appearance. He spoke only occasionally—mostly of self-blame for the way he treated his family business. He became afraid that he was going to die but refused to go to the hospital because he believed that the doctors there would tell him that he had a terminal illness.

He eventually consented to see the crisis therapist, who referred him to a psychiatrist for hospitalization. Isaac's history revealed that he was a small businessman who had done reasonably well but was always insecure and self-effacing. Several months prior to the exacerbation and onset of his condition, his business began to do poorly. As he was trying to cope with this business reversal his father died suddenly and unexpectedly of a heart attack. He grieved deeply and at the same time started to reproach himself for causing the family business to suffer. He progressively worsened to the point that he believed he had caused his father's death. When he began to speak of not being worthy of living, his wife called the crisis center.

The progressive development of Judy's depression, insomnia, and poor concentration, etc., suggest a clinical depression. Contrary to depression in crisis, Judy exhibits a history of long-standing depressive characteristics: low self-esteem, pessimistic attitude, feelings of inadequacy. As a general rule the individual in crisis may have the same symptoms, but the symptoms are only temporary in nature and are brought about by the inability to solve problems created by the precipitating event. In clinical depression the precipitating event exacerbates a pre-existing condition which the individual has been struggling with for months or years. For this person the precipitating event is truly the straw that broke the camel's back.

As far as clinical depression is concerned, Judy's case was a comparatively mild one, perhaps fitting the DSM-III (Diagnostic and Statistical Manual, American Psychiatric Association) classification of dysthymic disorder.

Isaac represents the more serious degree of depression, that is, a major depressive episode. In such severe cases of depression, referral to a psychiatrist is generally necessary.

As we have seen from the cases of Judy and Isaac, the seriousness of depression is determined by the level of psychosocial functioning and whether hospitalization is necessary. An important point is that clinical depression is generally precipitated by the same event that precipitates a crisis—namely, (a) a significant loss, of a loved one, self-esteem, emotional support, or psychosocial needs and roles; (b) failures, whether personal, economic, family, or occupational; (c) significant changes that threaten feelings of adequacy, competency, or performance. A major difference, however, is that in clinical depression there is a personality predisposition that is exacerbated by the precipitating event. The patient has a history of depressive characteristics that have interfered with maximum psychosocial functioning. When the precipitating event occurs, an even lower level of functioning results. The individual who is a pure crisis case has no history of clinical depression, and the depression results from the inability to solve the problem precipitated by the event; in clinical depression the precipitating event *reactivates* premorbity. In addition, the person in crisis resumes a normal level of functioning after crisis therapy, whereas in clinical depression the individual may or may not return to his or her maximum level of psychosocial functioning after prolonged therapy.

A Note on Depression and Anger

If the depressed person is also angry, he or she generally feels the anger to be basically unacceptable in some form. Consequently some feelings of guilt or unjustification for being angry will be present. This is because the depressed person generally has difficulty expressing anger outwardly, perhaps because he or she feels that a person who is angry is not lovable. Consequently the individual, for fear of not being loved or not being nice, turns the anger inward rather than expressing it directly at the object or person causing the frustration or deprivation (e.g., a loved one or an enemy).

It follows that, generally, the depressed person cannot express anger openly to an external source. If one could express anger, one would not become depressed. This does not mean, as is so popularly stated, that the therapist should routinely force the depressed person to express the anger. It should be remembered that the depressed person feels guilty about the anger, and turning it inward is a form of self-punishment. The depressed person is already experiencing the "bad me" role for the angry feelings, so to force the individual to express angry feelings before self-esteem has improved only reinforces the "bad" self-concept the person is currently experiencing. Sometimes giving permission to express anger to a person who is reluctant to do so may result in an excessive expression of anger. Therapeutic use of anger is discussed in Chapter 6. In the meantime it should suffice for therapists to recognize that sometimes the client will express anger toward them. Generally it is a subtle attack reflecting the client's expectation of the therapist's inability to help. This is often a reflection of the client's feeling of hopelessness; at other times it may be a test of the therapist's caring.

From this discussion of anxiety and depression, it is clear that the significance of the precipitating event to the person in crisis is reflected by whether the individual reacts with anxiety or depression. If the person reacts with anxiety, the precipitating event is perceived to be a threat to survival or welfare. If the person reacts with depression, the precipitating event represents a loss (e.g., love, self-esteem). Once the therapist determines whether the client is anxious or depressed, he or she can begin to ascertain why the precipitating event is perceived to have the significance it does. This can be determined by the client's communication, the subject of chapter 3.

REFERENCES

American Psychiatric Association. (1980). *Diagnostic and statistical manual of mental disorders* (DSM-III) (3rd ed.). Washington, D.C.: Author

Bibring, E. (1953) *The mechanism of depression.* In P. Greenacre (Ed.), *Affective disorders: Psychoanalytic contributions to this study.* New York: International Universities Press.

Bornstein, P. E., Clayton, P. J., Halikas, J. A., Maurice, W. I., & Robins, E. (1973). The depression of widowhood after thirteen months, *British Journal of Psychiatry, 122,* 561–566.

Bowlby, J. (1969). *Attachment: Vol. 1, Attachment and loss.* New York: Basic Books.

Bullard, D. M., Glaswer, H. H., Heagarty, M. C., & Pivchech, E. P. (1967). Failure to thrive in the neglected child. *American Journal of Orthopsychiatry, 37,* 680–690.

Dixon, S. L., & Sands, R. G. (1983). Identity and the experience of crisis, social casework. *The Journal of Contemporary Social Work, 9,* 13–140.

Erikson, E. H. (1963). *Childhood and society.* New York: W. W. Norton.

Freud, A. (1966). *The ego and the mechanisms of defense.* (Rev. ed.). New York: International Universities Press. (Originally published 1936).

Fromm-Reichmann, F. (1950) *Principles of intensive psychotherapy.* Chicago: University of Chicago Press.

Goldstein, A. P. (1962). *Therapist-patient expectations in psychotherapy.* New York: Macmillan.

Lamb, M. E. (1977). Father-infant and mother-infant interaction in the first year of life, *Child Development, 48,* 167–181.

Menninger, K., with Martin, M., & Pruyser, P. (1963). *The vital balance: The life process in mental health and illness,* New York: Viking Press.

Pemberton, D. A., & Benady, D. R. (1973). Consciously rejected children. *British Journal of Psychiatry, 123,* (576), 575–578.

Ribble, M. A. (1944). Infantile experience in relation to personality development. In J. McV. Hunt, (Ed.), *Personality and the behavior disorders* (vol. 2). New York: Ronald Press.

Rusk, T. N. (1971). Opportunity and techniques in crisis psychiatry. *Comprehensive Psychiatry, 12,*(3), 249–263.

Schachtel E. G. (1959). *Metamorphosis on the development of affect, perception, attention, and memory.* (p. 45). New York: Basic Books.

Spitz, R. A. (1945). *Hospitalism: An inquiry into the genesis of psychiatric conditions in early childhood; The psychoanalystic study of the child.* New York: International Universities Press, *1,* 53–74.

SUGGESTED READINGS

Davitz, J. R. (1959). Fear, anxiety and the perception of others. *Journal of General Psychology, 61,* 169–173.

Laughlin, H. P. (1970). *The ego and its defenses.* New York: Appleton-Century-Crofts.

May, R. (1950). *The meaning of anxiety.* New York: Ronald Press.

Mendels, J. (1970). *Concepts of depression.* New York: John Wiley & Sons.

Rochlin, G. R. (1959). The loss complex: A contribution to the etiology of depression. *Journal of the American Psychoanalytic Association, 7,* 299–316.

3

Communication Process in Crisis Intervention

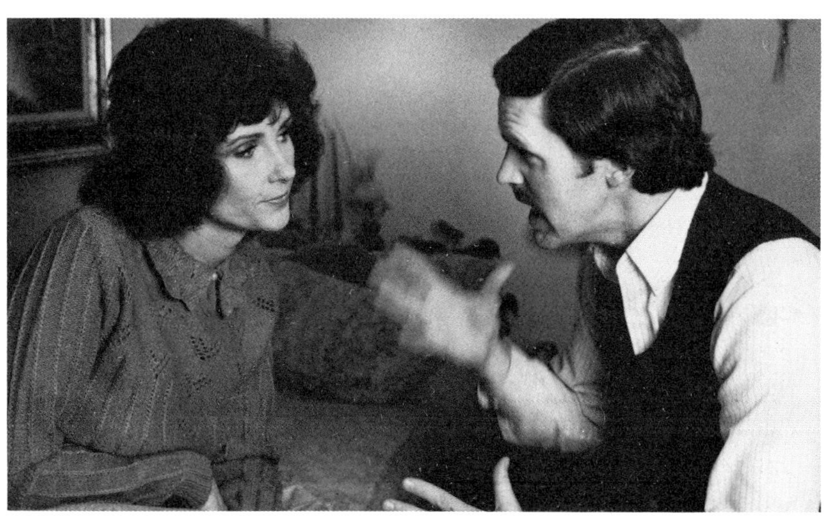

Therapist:	How are you feeling today?
Client:	Great, I got a job with a security company.
Therapist:	How does that feel?
Client:	At first I was nervous, it was a ritzy place. I thought they would only want a high quality person.
Therapist:	They hired you. How does it feel to be top quality?
Client:	Good. (*changes subject*) I saw my father this weekend. I went home to pick up more of my clothes.

This is a brief excerpt from the second interview of crisis therapy. It is easy to see how people communicate their feelings and attitudes about themselves and their world—their psychic reality. From this communication intervention we see that the client's self-concept is poor (I thought they only wanted high quality people) and that the therapist tried to enhance it too early (how does it feel to be top quality), which caused the client to reject the therapist's efforts (changes subject).

If crisis intervention is to have any value, the client must improve and change through the therapeutic relationship; that is, through interpersonal interactions with the therapist. The ways the client and therapist communicate determine the nature of the therapeutic relationship, and conversly the nature of the relationship affects the communication process. Hence the heart of learning how to work with people therapeutically is learning to communicate with them. Communication is the process through which clients convey their distress. It is the process through which the therapist implements his or her knowledge of human behavior. Most often the keys to therapeutic success or failure can be found in therapist-client communication. As a helping professional, the therapist should control the communication situation (even though this relationship is mutually determined, as all relationships are). Understanding the basics of interpersonal communication should increase the therapist's skills in helping people in crisis.

WHAT IS HUMAN COMMUNICATION?

Human beings are born with a capacity to communicate. We have inborn systems to transmit, receive, and process information, although the *ways* we do so are learned. Most of us learn to *encode* our meanings to transmit a message and to *decode* another person's messages to receive the meaning.

Let us now look at what communication is. For the purpose of this book, we can say that human communication is *the processes one individual uses to affect the behavior of another*. In our model, a *sender* is one who wants to influence another by sending some stimulus. The *receiver* is the one whom the sender wants to influence. Regardless of the seeming insignificance of the message, the basic goal of the sender remains the same: to influence the receiver. Each interpersonal communication "transaction" involves three elements: a sender, a message, and a receiver.

SENDER

Communication is a social interaction between two or more people in a specific social context. Within the specific context, the communication process starts with the sender, who first internally experiences some need to communicate. The sender wants to influence the receiver by sending a message; but to do so, signals or symbols must be used that both the sender and the intended receiver will understand. Words, gestures, or other symbols the sender believes will transmit the message most effectively must be selected. These words and gestures become the symbolic representations of the sender's feelings and experiences. Again, the sender encodes the message.

It seems as though choosing effective communication signals would be easy, and it can be when the message is clear, forthright, and unambiguous. But it is a problem in most human communication. The exact meaning the sender wants to communicate cannot be communicated as it was originally experienced inside the sender's head. Therefore the sender always takes the risk that the message might be misunderstood, that his or her purpose might not be achieved, or that the message might be rejected. The difficulty can occur when the real meaning of the message is unknown even to the sender, either because it has gotten lost in the encoding process or because some unconscious motivation interfered. In addition, the individual's idiosyncratic psychic system—the ways he or she has learned to act toward other people—affects how messages are encoded and what is chosen to communicate. When the client is the sender and the therapist is the receiver, the sender's real goal—to influence another person—must always be at the forefront of the therapist's mind.

Even before a thought, feeling, or impulse is transmitted as a message, it passes through a series of internal screens. Most people give a great deal of thought to a message before they send it. They try to shape a message in a way most likely to get the desired response. Even as young children we learn that we are not likely to reach our communication goals unless we transmit messages in ways acceptable to ourselves and others. These ways may not be the exact translations of our feelings. The original message may be antisocial, hostile, self-centered, or otherwise socially unacceptable. Therefore we learn to encode the original message into symbols or behavior we believe will achieve the desired goals. If the sender believes that a message will be rejected or will work to his or her disadvantage, he or she will not express it directly or clearly, but will disguise it.

By the time people reach adulthood, they have developed internal screens that prevent them from transmitting emotionally unacceptable thoughts, feelings, and ideas. These screens may be used consciously or unconsciously. Many messages never get encoded because of anticipated consequences. Certain words or feelings, such as curse words or extreme jealously, may be completely blocked and never encoded.

FACTORS AFFECTING COMMUNICATION

Once a person decides it is appropriate to express a feeling or idea, he or she must select and transmit symbols for that experience. One can choose words, language, affect, gestures, postures, and other behavioral manifestations as symbols. To understand the meaning of the message, the receiver needs to know not only the meaning of the words but also their usage and form within the language. Because most of our daily communication is accomplished with relatively few familiar words, most people assume that words and language mean the same thing to everybody. But they do not. Communication symbols are only substitutes for reality; they are not the reality itself. The specific ways a person communicates are determined by several significant factors.

First and foremost are the specific life experiences of the individual—the ways the individual has been socialized. Most newborn infants have the capacity to interact with their environment through biological reflex action. For instance, they cry when they are in pain. These biological reflex actions are given a meaning by the caretaker (e.g., the mother smoothes powder on the baby's chafed skin). Thus the infant begins to learn that reactions can be provoked from the external world. Eventually the baby learns to associate words and language with specific experiences and then with groups of experiences. "Milk" is not just the liquid in this cup; it is the liquid I drank yesterday and will drink tonight. Not only is language developed in this fashion, but people learn to meet needs and to negotiate the environment in this way.

Each human being's life is a continuity of experiences, and individual methods of communication reflect those experiences. Each word contains all the associations accumulated to date. Hence individuals from different cultures, subcultures, and even different neighborhoods will have different frames of reference and, therefore, different communication patterns. One important topic currently receiving a great deal of attention by linguists is minority communication patterns such as "black language," the idiosyncratic rules of grammar and meanings of English used by many blacks. For example, many blacks use and understand the expression, "Sometimes it bes' that way." To translate that statement into edited American English we would say, "That is the way life is sometimes; that is reality and it is unchanging: accept it and do not worry about it." That underlying meaning would be unknown to someone unfamiliar with the American black subculture. The therapist who wishes to communicate with a member of a subculture must learn to "speak the language."

A second factor that determines the way one communicates is the social context in which the communication occurs. Most people communicate differently in a formal setting than in an informal one. For example, you use different language to express frustration in the office than on the tennis court.

A third factor that determines how a person communicates is the roles of those communicating. For example, students generally communicate differently with their professors than with each other. Clients generally communicate differently with therapists than with peers. Roles and status are important in therapy situations because they can provoke feelings about authority and self-images.

This leads to the fourth factor that contributes to the way each person communicates: self-concept. *Self-concept* is how individuals see themselves and their own identities. It involves perception, real and imagined personality, abilities, and weaknesses. Most individuals communicate most of the time in ways consistent with their self-concepts. Remember, communication involves both transmitting and receiving. People not only transmit information in ways consistent with their self-concept (be it positive or negative), but they also receive information that way. In fact, much communication is designed to enhance, maintain, or defend one's self-concept as well as to reflect it. Thus a great deal of receptive communication is influenced by whether the receiver perceives the message as a threat to his or her own self-concept. However, most people are largely unaware of their feelings about themselves and therefore are unaware of much of what they communicate. Whether recognized or not, self-concept is reflected by an individual's communication patterns. For example, negative self-concepts may be reflected when people neglect themselves or are unassertive or allow themselves to be exploited. Superior self-concepts can be reflected in habits of talking down to people or in using complicated words and phrases to impress or dramatize.

Self-concept influences perception of others as well. The basis for perceiving others is directly related to how people perceive themselves.

A fifth factor is education. This factor can be very important when people with different amounts or kinds of education communicate, especially if the person with more education does not take this difference into consideration. It is important that the more highly educated person not look down on the other, but that he or she choose words and phrases that are common, clear, and easily understood. The skill of a therapist can be determined by how effectively he or she translates theory and certain concepts into words understandable by all, regardless of educational level.

A sixth factor in determining how one person communicates with another is previous experience with the same person. People who communicate frequently learn each other's habitual patterns, feelings, and preferences. When people are familiar with each other, they can take shortcuts; they can make assumptions about the other's responses. For instance, a student may say, "To get a good grade, you must say what Professor O'Connell wants to hear." The student is simply saying that he or she has already learned something about the professor. Many clients learn very quickly to say what they think the therapist wants to hear, or to say what is socially expected.

RECEIVER

Thus far we have been discussing communication from the viewpoint of the sender. But the *consequence* of the communication process is determined by how the receiver interprets the sender's message, since that is what will determine the receiver's reaction. Once the sender transmits the message, he or she loses control over it. Communication is a process of cumulative social interaction. The receiver goes through a process similar to that of the sender. But what determines the way the receiver responds to the communication symbols—to the sender's words, language, tone of voice, nonverbal gestures? How does predisposition influence the way one reacts? The emotional disposition of the receiver and the experiences associated with the symbols chosen by the sender determine the reaction.

Consider the communication system of the receiver. Reception is no less complicated than transmission. Each receiver also has a set of mental barriers and screens that control not only what is heard, but how it is heard. People screen various stimuli in all communication, partially because there are too many stimuli (words, voice, movement, facial expression, hands) to attend to them all. They consciously and unconsciously select certain stimuli to which they will respond and omit others. Through this weeding-out process the meaning of the message can be changed. The receiver may be protected by being on guard against messages that make him or her feel anxious and uncomfortable or that disturb self-perception or self-esteem. For example, a woman who prides herself on being well liked may be greatly upset by someone telling her that her friends do not like her when she talks too much. And she may choose to ignore the message, interpreting it as a sign of the sender's hostility or jealously toward her. Most people have internal needs that result from the development of their own unique psychic systems and lead to particular sensitivity to certain stimuli.

Another factor that influences what people hear is self-interest. People generally hear those things that interest or stimulate them, that affect their own welfare, or that meet their needs or expectations, either positive or negative. Some people are "set" to hear negative things about themselves, especially if they think negatively about themselves. On the other hand, they will ignore or misinterpret those positive messages that threaten their internal consistency. Just as the sender has motives for initiating the communication, the receiver has motives and attitudes that facilitate reception of certain stimuli and avoidance of others.

Certain defense mechanisms (see chapter 2) play an important part in what one hears. For example, a person who is projecting may hear what he or she would have said rather than what actually was said. In reaction formation, the opposite of what was actually said is heard; in the use of repression and denial, the message is not heard at all. These defense mechanisms, so inherent in our mental processes, affect the degree of accuracy with which a message is received. They protect people from hearing things that would be inconvenient, harmful, or anxiety producing.

Expectation is another factor that influences reception. People often hear what they expect to hear, whether it is said or not. Sometimes they do this because they have a stereotyped idea of a group to which the sender belongs. For instance, a person with a shaggy beard and long hair may be expected to express radical ideas. A woman lawyer may be expected to be conservative. The tendency to attribute to individuals the characteristics of the group with whom they are associated is widespread, and often what is heard is what a person is expected to say rather than what is said. Professional therapists need to understand the various groups with whom they work and look beyond the groups to individual people.

Process of Reception

Any stimulus or message from a sender travels to a receiver; the receiver uses some sense organs, usually the eyes and the ears, to take in the stimulus. The stimulus is transmitted to the brain, and the message is psychologically received. Then the process of decoding begins. The receiver interprets the message, making it consistent with his or her frame of reference. Again, each receiver has a unique frame of reference determined by his or her life experiences, self-concept, level of education, status in the relationship, and the social context. At times, a message may remind a receiver (especially one under stress) of a previous similar situation that may or may not have any relevance. The receiver may compare the old and new situations and translate the current one according to previous perceptions. In so doing, the receiver may distort the current messages by omitting some information and modifying certain ideas to make them acceptable or justifiable, thus responding to a different message than the sender intended. If the sender then responds to the distorted perceptions, that response may also be inappropriate.

SUCCESSFUL COMMUNICATION

The full meaning of the form and content of any communication interaction cannot be understood without considering both the sender and the receiver. When both feel they have benefited, a communication exchange is successful. But it is not easy to succeed. Let us look at why.

First, both the sender and the receiver have some goal in the communication exchange. The receiver's first response to the sender's first message begins a cumulative social interaction. Both the sender and receiver usually want to benefit from the exchange, which may lead to significant differences and disagreements if both don't achieve their communication goals.

Second, communication involves symbols, both verbal and nonverbal. While a fist to the eye is a pretty direct method of expression, even it is open to interpretation. And language is much less specific—much more open to the meaning each person brings to it. To better understand how language contributes to difficulties in communicating, we must look more closely at the nature of language itself.

Meaning of Language

We use language to represent reality, but it can never be the reality itself. A language is a system of symbols that a social group uses to communicate. The members of the group agree on both specific symbols to represent specific ideas or objects—*words*—and rules for stringing those symbols together—*syntax*. Language is only a substitute for the reality that it attempts to represent, and reality is actually much more complex than the meaning language can convey. For example, we call a four-legged, furry animal with a wagging tail and certain other characteristics simply a dog, and as long as everyone shares this understanding, communication can take place. The meaning of the word "dog" is arbitrarily assigned by the group of people who speak English. We could easily call this animal something else, perhaps *chien*, as the French do. The point is simply that the meaning of the word must be understood by everyone in the social group. Those who do not understand the common meaning cannot communicate.

However, the process of communication is not made simple by the sharing of a common language; there are not enough words in any language to give an exact representation of all shades of ideas, feelings, and experiences. Words call into play feelings and memories associated with previous experiences. To some people, "dog" has a very specific meaning; to someone who has never owned a dog, the word conveys less information than to someone who has, and still other information is conveyed to someone who has been bitten by a dog. The meaning a word evokes for a receiver may be based on experience with the symbol and with the referent itself.

In other words, using the same language is only half of the communication process. Experience gives language meaning. Each individual's perceptions, emotions, and thoughts come from experiences; language represents these experiences, and the experiences give meaning to the language. Thus communication is facilitated through common experiences. People in low socioeconomic groups and those in the middle socioeconomic groups may have difficulty understanding each other because of different life experiences and different goals and values. For instance, the word "hunger" will have a different meaning for someone who has actually faced not having enough to eat than for someone who gets "hungry" an hour before each meal. Those two people may have trouble communicating about the problem of a lost job if they do not understand their differences. It is important to remember that *experiences,* not class memberships, are the major differences between two individuals. Although a great deal is made over racial and cultural differences, it is personal *experiences* that should be the basis for understanding. Individual members of racial and ethnic minorities may have had the same experiences as the majority group. The romantic experiences of two white Anglo-Saxon teenagers, one healthy and one with cerebral palsy, may be more different from each other than from those of the healthy teenager and Chicano counterparts. Expectations and stereotyping should not be allowed to intrude into the communication process. Each exchange should start where the two participants are, not where each thinks the other is.

In most communication situations, the sender and the receiver assume that they are on the same frequency and that they both understand the words used. This often is not true, and communication fails. How many times have you said, "I did not mean it that way" or "That was not what I said"? Thus, for communication to be successful, both parties must choose their language carefully, considering all those factors we have discussed: the background of the other person, the status relationships, the specific situation, and educational background.

Language is problematic because it is composed of symbols that are emotionally laden, have multiple meanings, and represent memories of experiences and not the experiences themselves.

The weakness of language as a communication medium is not cause for alarm. Functionally, language has a broader purpose than mere social interaction; it is a tool we use to describe, understand, and control the environment and extend it beyond our own physical capacities. We understand certain ideas only because we have language to describe them, not because we have personal experience with them.

Meaning of Words

The basis of any language is an oral system; the basic unit is the spoken word. In everyday speech, most of us use a relatively limited familiar vocabulary that we take for granted. The words become so familiar that we may think that the words we use are real themselves, that they are not simply arbitrary sounds. But words *are* arbitrary; they are symbols representing experiences and feelings and are loaded with old emotions and experiences.

It is on this basis that words have a great capacity to evoke strong feelings. For example, words such as "macho," "equality," "libber," and "freedom" can provoke equally strong but widely varying meanings in different people and under different conditions. For example, the familiar word "independence" can be a very powerful emotional stimulus for adolescents attempting to emancipate themselves from their parents. Some words are so powerfully emotive that responses to people may be irrational. The words "busing" and "strike," for example, have become quite powerful. "Busing" only recently achieved this power, in spite of the fact that children have been riding buses to school for generations. But today, to many people, "busing" can mean poor education, mixing the races, wasting money, and fear.

Other taboo words have enormous emotional power and control over people's behavior and feelings. Magical and superstitious powers are attributed to certain words used in rituals and ceremonies. Words can make rational and logical people think and behave illogically. They can be used for deliberate deception or for arousing prejudices of all kinds.

For the therapist, words can reduce emotional upset and restore the client's cognitive control. Words can evoke strong emotions because a person has fused the word with what it represents in the mind. Words with double meanings, or overly emotive words, are more likely to have strong personal interpretations, which decreases the chances the sender's message will be understood. The therapist should remember this and carefully choose words with the client's individual life experiences, educational level, and social context in mind. Understanding how words can evoke powerful feelings is a critical skill for the therapist. In fact, words and language are the non-medical therapist's most important tools.

Denotative and Connotative Meanings of Words

A second difficulty with words (in addition to their emotional power) is their multiple meanings. Words have two types of meanings: denotative and connotative. Denotative meanings are the literal meanings—the dictionary definition of a word on which all users of the language agree.

Some words have more than one denotative meaning. For instance, the word "class" can mean a group of items ranked together possessing common characteristics, or it can mean a group of people brought together for the purpose of education. A university student, asked to which class he or she belongs, may not be sure whether the question refers to educational level, economic status, or social background. Miscommunication can be the result.

The connotative meaning of a word involves all the word's associations and emotional meanings. Again take "class" as an example. In addition to denoting a group, it can have the connotative meaning of "refinement": "She has class." The ordinary words "pig" and "turkey" have recently taken on negative connotative meaning. Connotations can be given to a word by a small subgroup of a population and offer another hurdle in the path of successful communication between therapist and client. For instance, the therapist unfamiliar with the current connotation of "turkey" might respond inappropriately to being called one.

Nonverbal Communication

Nonverbal messages are transmitted by behaviors other than speech. They include gestures, facial expressions, posture, body movements, tone of voice and intonation, and, quite frequently, dress. Nonverbal messages can occur in conjunction with verbal communication and are often used to reinforce verbal communication (consider a greeting such as a handshake, for example; even the strength of the handshake can be significant). But nonverbal messages can be and often are independent of verbal communication (consider the person who looks at a watch every five minutes during a conversation). A combination of consistent verbal and nonverbal messages produces the clearest communication.

Generally, nonverbal messages are easily interpreted and have meanings that are often determined by social context. Gestures that occur most often along with speech include head and hand movements. They are often used for emphasis; examples include pointing and tracing an object with the hands. Facial expressions are used to show emotions such as happiness, anger, surprise, fear, sadness, or frustration. Head and hand movements are probably the most frequently used methods of nonverbal communication and are often used by people who have difficulty expressing their ideas or feelings verbally. Gestures expressing anger, such as frowning, are easily interpreted. The angry motorist shaking a fist is another example.

Body posture and movement can also reflect feelings; it can indicate interest and enthusiasm or boredom. Posture can indicate anxiety (consider the person poised on the edge of a chair) or depression. It can indicate joy as well.

Nonverbal communication is important largely because both the sender and the receiver are greatly influenced by what they see. They interpret the meaning of nonverbal messages personally, just as they do verbal messages. The sender's nonverbal cues advise the receiver of the proper response to the message, and the sender uses the receiver's nonverbal clues to gauge the reception of the message. A nod of the head and an attentive facial expression communicate to a speaker that a member of the audience is interested in the speech.

Many people are unaware of the nonverbal messages they send. These messages may be inconsistent with the person's verbal behavior. For instance, Diana, an attractive woman, complained tearfully that men were always making passes at her. She felt they were thinking she was "available." Diana had grown up in a strict home in which any form of seductiveness was severely admonished. Thus she had repressed her curiosity about this behavior. But even though it had always been forbidden, she had feelings that led her to dress and move in ways that men found attractive. She unconsciously communicated seductive behavior nonverbally. The fact that men responded made her feel guilty, although she was unaware of her seductive behavior. But the therapist could see the inconsistency in Diana's verbal messages and her nonverbal signal.

There are times that tone of voice, intonation, and speed of speech are also nonverbal communication. They are especially meaningful when they are inconsistent with the meaning of the verbal message. When this occurs, their nonverbal meaning is generally a more accurate reflection of feelings. This is discussed further in chapter 4.

THE THERAPIST'S ROLE IN THE COMMUNICATION PROCESS

When learning to work with people in crisis we need to devote special attention to the therapist's style of communicating. The therapist's contribution to the communication process is the ability to listen to both verbal and nonverbal messages in order to understand cognitively and empathetically what the client is experiencing and saying in the confusion of the crisis. The therapist must be able to convey meaningfully to the client what the client feels, and at the same time provide an understanding of the client's chaos and confusion. If self-understanding (cognitive restoration) is a factor in crisis reduction and improved functioning, it can only be achieved through the therapist's ability to communicate in a way the client can understand and find meaningful. McCarthy and Knapp (1984) studied the helping styles of three groups of therapists: crisis interveners, psychotherapists, and untrained individuals. They wanted to ascertain whether crisis interveners were more active and leading than psychotherapists—whether crisis interveners actually responded more often and used more questions, advice, influence, and information. They hypothesized that psychotherapists would be more empathetic and non-directive than either crisis interveners or untrained individuals, responding less frequently and utilizing reflections of client content and affect more often. The researchers found that crisis interveners were active and directive; the psychotherapists were less leading and more empathetic. Untrained subjects did more talking than listening and quickly jumped to conclusions with little problem exploration.

Although McCarthy and Knapp did not study the relative effectiveness of each group, it appears that the most effective crisis therapist is one who combines dimensions of the crisis intervener and the psychotherapist: active and directive, or empathetic and insight-oriented, as the situation dictates (Hobbs, 1984). The important point is to understand that however one intervenes, it is the communication process that should be the focus of study and learning.

The therapist's style of communicating is influenced by his or her theoretical position, as well a factor influencing the client such as education, life experiences, perception, and self-concept. One of the therapist's primary tasks is to understand the client through the client's communication process.

SUMMARY

Communication is a process of social interaction in which people attempt to influence each other to achieve some more or less specific goal.

Although communication occurs on all levels, true communication can take place only when there is understanding and agreement between the persons involved. Human communication is based on the transmission and reception of stimuli consisting of verbal and nonverbal symbols having predetermined meanings. Communication's success is determined by the accuracy of the receiver's interpretation of the intended meaning of the sender's message. Messages are encoded and decoded according to life experiences, including culture, education, and socioeconomic status, and according to each individual's psychic system. Clear communication occurs when a stimulus is encoded and transmitted freely and clearly and decoded in such a way that the receiver accurately interprets the meaning. Although it may be easier to communicate with those who share similar experiences, almost any two people have some areas of common understanding that can serve as a primary focus in all communication.

The importance of understanding the communication process cannot be overemphasized. It is especially important to understand the cumulative interactive nature of the communication process, the meaning and evocative capacities of words and language, and the importance of nonverbal communication. In crisis communication, the clients' messages, feelings, and ideas may be confusing even to themselves, and they may not be aware of what they want to communicate. The ability of the therapist to hear and interpret a client's messages and provide feedback is a most important tool. The therapist must keep in mind the client's crisis state and interpret and respond according to knowledge of human behavior. A person in crisis is experiencing a variety of painful and confusing feelings. The therapist must be able to sort out these feelings and communicate them back to the client in such a way that the client can understand what is occurring within himself or herself. The client then receives, digests, translates, and interprets the meaning of the therapist's messages and again responds. Thus the interaction perpetuates itself. If the client feels understood, accepted, and respected, regardless of the crisis condition or behavior, a good relationship will result. For both the client and therapist, the willingness to continue to communicate depends on the hope that positive benefits will result to each person involved. When this is no longer believed to be possible, efforts to communicate stop.

Chapter 4 is devoted to the application of this basic model of communication to the process and techniques of therapeutic intervention, especially the initial interview.

REFERENCES

Hobbs, M. (1984). Crisis intervention in theory and practice: A selected review. *British Journal of Medical Psychology, 57,* 23–34.

McCarthy, P. R., & Knapp, S. L. (1984). Helping Styles of Crisis Interveners, Psychotherapists, and Untrained Individuals. *American Journal of Community Psychology, 12,* (3).

SUGGESTED READINGS

Cherry, C. (1978). *On human communication.* New York: John Wiley & Sons.

Kadushin, A. (1972). *The social work interview.* New York: Columbia University Press.

4

Process and Techniques of Crisis Intervention

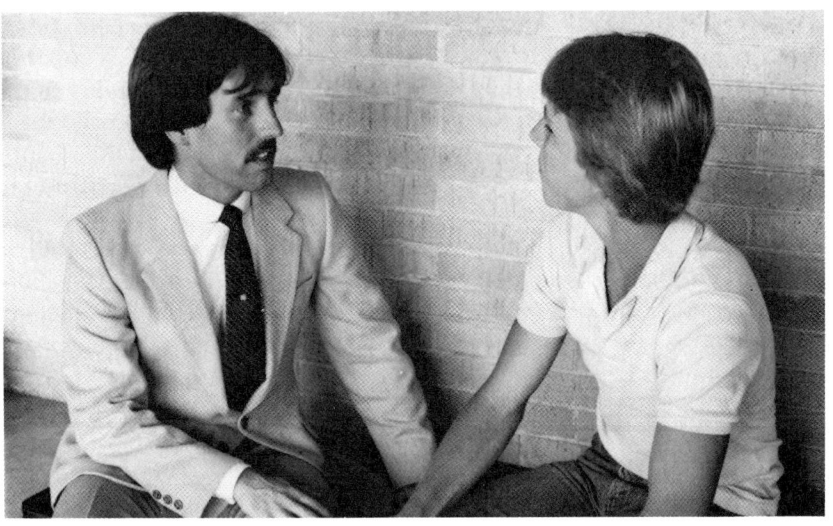

Case Studies

Quentin, a 32-year-old single man, came to the crisis center depressed and talking of suicide. The day before coming, he had broken up with a woman he had been dating for more than a year. He was tearful as he spoke of this relationship as the longest he had ever had. Although he realized that this woman was special to him, he could not understand his reaction to the breakup since he had broken off many relationships in the past.

Theresa, a 28-year-old married mother, came to the crisis center depressed and guilt ridden over an abortion she had had five days earlier. Her husband had just taken a new job in another state when they learned she was pregnant. Although she wanted to have the baby, she had the abortion to please her husband. She now felt guilty about it, believing she had committed an unpardonable sin by taking a human life. Because of her depression and guilt, she felt unable to join her husband.

Bill, age 40, a successful executive, came to the crisis center on the insistence of his doctor, who could find no organic reasons for Bill's complaints that he was having a heart attack. Bill had become "very emotional" since receiving a promotion and substantial salary increase. By the third day on his new job, he had become so anxious he had to go home. At home he was jittery, paced the floor, complained that he did not know what was wrong, and that he felt apprehensive, as if something terrible were going to happen to him. As his anxiety became worse, he began to feel as if he were going to die of a heart attack.

These case examples illustrate that crisis is a time of emotional disturbance and cognitive disorganization, and that a wide range of individuals can experience crisis regardless of previous level of psychosocial functioning, socio-economic status, or history of psychopathology. When working with such a diverse client population, we must remember that the nature of the person experiencing the crisis is as important as the precipitating event. In order to help people like Quentin, Theresa, and Bill, we must first understand their personalities, since each precipitating event has a subjective meaning for the individual that we can understand only by coming to know the person and his or her frame of reference. For instance, what personal meanings did Quentin attach to the breakup of his romance, and Theresa to her abortion? Why did Bill experience a promotion depression at this time in his life? What makes him feel undeserving of success and fearful of failure? Are the meanings to be found in the client's past or present? Do these meanings threaten the reactivation of some unconscious conflict?

The first three chapters of this book presented information to help us gain a theoretical understanding of psychosocial functioning and behavior of people in crisis. Based on this theoretical knowledge, this chapter provides the process and techniques for helping people in crisis to reduce the crippling effect of emotionality, anxiety, anger, and depression. Through the use of cognitive restructuring techniques, personality growth can occur. Viney, Clarke, Bum and Benjamin (1985) state that "... crisis intervention counseling also strikes deeper to restructure personality and thus produce growth ... This involves clients using insight into their past, not only to resolve the current crisis, but to establish ways to minimize failure and to adapt to potential crisis in the future ..."

THE PROCESS OF CRISIS THERAPY

In crisis therapy, there is a general sequential process or course of crisis intervention, which may vary with some people and situations but usually remains the same. Understanding this process enables the therapist to be aware of what he or she is doing or should be doing at any given time.

Crisis therapy begins when a client seeks help for a significant problem that the client cannot solve. It is understood that between the time of the occurrence of the event that precipitated the crisis and the first intervention, the client has been trying to solve the problem alone. This fact is important because it determines how the client appears at the first interview. At the first interview, the client may either (a) manifest one or more of the common crisis reactions: high emotionalism, tension, anxiety, depression, anger, and so forth, or (b) submerge or hold back intense emotionalism generally associated with a crisis, manifesting only the effect of the emotionalism; that is, feelings of helplessness and inability to take action. The client may also express fear, worry, and concern. In these cases, focusing on the precipitating event(s), specifically the feelings, meaning, and circumstances surrounding it, will generally reactivate characteristics of emotionalism. In this stage of the process, the nature of the relationship has become significant as the client experiences the therapist's attentiveness, concern, empathy, acceptance, and understanding.

While exploring the facts, feelings, and meaning associated with the precipitating event, the therapist listens on two levels: (a) to what clients actually say and (b) to the meaning of what clients say. The task here is to begin gathering information leading to the nuclear problem—the unconscious meaning of the problem caused by the precipitating event. Consider, for example, the following case:

> Ann, a 35-year-old woman, came to a mental health agency distraught, depressed, and feeling helpless after her husband told her he thought he wanted a divorce and that he wanted to go away for a while to make up his mind. Initially, Ann cried profusely, stating that she did not know what she was going to do, and that she felt she could not live without her husband. She confessed that the pain of losing her husband was so great she thought she could not go on living. The therapist acknowledged silently that this was a painful situation but noted that Ann's husband had not actually divorced her and wondered why she was reacting as if he already had.
>
> Further explanation revealed that Ann's father had left her mother and her about the time her mother was her age and Ann was about eight. Both Ann and her mother experienced intense emotional pain for a long time afterward, her mother even talking of suicide.

In the case of Ann, we see that past experience can make one vulnerable and sensitive to the threat of a present loss. Under the circumstances, Ann was unable to deal with her present problem because she perceived it from the experience of a previous unresolved loss. More specifically, Ann's nuclear problem related to the fact that she never dealt with her father leaving her and her mother some 27 years before.

Following the evaluation and discovery of the nuclear problem, the therapist should provide the client with feedback regarding what the client is experiencing, what causes it, and why. A treatment plan should then be offered along with a concise course of action for the client. At this point, the therapist also should furnish the client with hope and optimism, always being careful, however, not to promise more than can be achieved.

The initial interview should generate a great deal of client trust. Generally, people in crisis regain a substantial amount of their cognitive functioning and equilibrium after discussing the precipitating event and exploring the emotionalism associated with it. The second phase of intervention primarily involves discussing current feelings, behavior, and action taken since the initial interview. After this second phase, the therapist should notice a change in perception, problem definition, and consequences; the client's strengths and assets should begin to become apparent to the client. In the third phase, greater use is made of cognitive restoration techniques, and greater interpretation of nuclear problem involvement can occur. When the debilitating effects of the precipitating event have diminished, and an effective level of psychosocial functioning has been achieved, termination of crisis therapy is indicated. In the fourth phase, termination is discussed: loose ends are tied together, major strengths are emphasized, procedures for handling future problems are reviewed, and plans for follow-up are established. Now, let us study the techniques of crisis interviewing, and later, the techniques of crisis intervention.

THE THERAPEUTIC INTERVIEW

As we saw in chapter 3, communication is crucial to the therapeutic relationship and, as such, is the foundation for interviewing. From that base, this chapter discusses a most important skill: therapeutic interviewing. Special attention is given to the first interview, since it is the most crucial factor in determining a therapist's ability to help a client resolve a crisis. Errors in subsequent sessions generally do not affect the outcome as much as those in the first session.

Although crisis therapy may take place anywhere (on a street, on a bridge, on the telephone, in an emergency room of a hospital, in a home, or in an office), the process of interviewing and treatment are basically the same, given circumstantial variations. The interventive process and techniques in this chapter are not limited to crisis therapy; however, in working with people in crisis they are used much more actively and rapidly. Consequently their use in crisis therapy requires considerable understanding and skill.

Preinterview Factors

Even before the first interview begins, the relationship is affected by several factors having to do with both the client and the therapist. The first is that the client is asking the therapist for help. Even though the client in crisis is more helpless and more amenable to being helped than at any other time in life, his or her feelings and attitudes about asking for emotional help should be considered. Even though society's attitude toward asking for help has greatly improved, many people still feel anxious about it. Many clients delay seeking help for some time, not only because they are trying to solve their problems themselves but also because of their reluctance to ask for help. This is exemplified by Deborah, who came for help after ineffectively struggling for several weeks with her grief over the sudden and unexpected death of Bob, her husband. She had talked for about an hour and had begun to feel better when she suddenly said, "I'm sorry I had to come; Bob would not have wanted me to be here. He would have considered it a sign of weakness, and he always wanted me to be strong." A client's negative feelings about seeking help should be dealt with, since they generally reflect the client's pride and perhaps self-concept. Therefore they may be obstacles to therapeutic goals.

A second preinterview factor is the therapist's confidence—the self-assurance that he or she will be able to help the client. This is of particular concern to new therapists. Self-awareness and confrontation of self-doubts or possibly harmful feelings will go a long way toward reducing their effect. However, experience is the best long-term cure.

A third preinterview condition worth noting is initial perception—the impressions gained from first sight to the beginning of the official interview. For better or for worse, people form impressions from the ways other people look, act, and talk before getting to know them. We let new stimuli reactivate previous images, impressions, and experiences to give us some control over new and unfamiliar situations. It is not unusual for a client to look at the therapist and match the therapist's appearance or physical characteristics with those of someone in the client's past. Or the client may initially feel that a therapist is warm or cold on the basis of some personal characteristics. Such initial impressions are an inevitable part of being human, of the effort to make the unfamiliar familiar. Therapists should strive to be sincere and to be themselves in their choice of dress and behavior. But dress should not be so different from the professional norm that it becomes an obstacle. Nor should initial behavior be out of line with the norm. Preinterview conditions can either facilitate the communication process and the establishment of a therapeutic relationship, or conditions can retard them. The therapist's first task is to be aware of them.

THE PROCESS OF INTERVIEWING

The initial therapeutic interview has two purposes: to begin development of a shared feeling of understanding and to assess the client's condition and social functioning so the therapist can help resolve the crisis. Sharing means the client will learn about his or her own condition through the interaction. The crisis therapist must quickly ascertain information that leads to an understanding and an assessment of the client's problems, condition, and level of social functioning. The process of interviewing is the major medium by which these goals are achieved.

It should be clear by now that the interaction between therapist and client is the means through which the client benefits and constructive changes occur. The communication process is the heart of the therapeutic intervention, and it depends on the relationship between therapist and client. Thus the first task in therapeutic interviewing is to establish a constructive relationship. Let us look at how this can be achieved.

The Therapeutic Relationship

Because the therapeutic relationship is so important to therapeutic outcome, the crisis therapist must know as much as possible about it. It differs from a social relationship. The goals of social relationships are fun, mutual stimulation, and satisfaction. The purpose of the therapeutic relationship is to alleviate the client's problems and improve social functioning. It is a relationship that promotes emotional growth and learning. The client is not expected to gratify the therapist's social and psychological needs. The many amenities of social relationships are omitted from the therapeutic relationship and the resolution of the client's problem is always in the therapist's mind. Sometimes, light social behavior is believed to be the basis of a good relationship. But a client in crisis is unhappy; he or she is suffering emotionally. Light social behavior may make the client feel that his or her problems are not being taken seriously or that he or she is not important. This does not mean there is no place for humor in a therapeutic relationship, but the therapist must resist the temptation to avoid the client's distress by making light and nonserious conversation. Regardless of the possible humor, this is not the time to say, "It is better laughed about" or "At least you can still laugh about it."

Establishing a Therapeutic Relationship

At the start of the official first interview, the therapist should be aware of the preinterview conditions as part of the observation procedure. However, these are preliminary; most often the beginning of the real relationship starts with the first official contact with the client in the office or other therapeutic setting. In cases where first contact between client and therapist is by telephone, the communication and relationship start then. Telephone communication tends to increase the importance of the preinterview conditions. In such cases, characteristics of a therapeutic relationship are just as operable as in face-to-face situations.

The success or failure of the entire therapeutic process can depend on the opening of the first interview. The therapist should behave seriously, being neither unduly light nor overly friendly. Greetings should be in keeping with personality, but genuinely warm and cordial, in a natural, quite tone. Overly friendly, loud welcomings should be avoided. Sullivan (1954) states that although he does not overwelcome clients, he does try to convey that they were expected and that he wished to see them. The client should be greeted by title and last name. The use of first names should never be taken for granted. If the therapist prefers first names, their use should be delayed until the client and therapist know and feel comfortable with each other. Using first-name greetings before a good relationship has been established can cause a problem for some clients; they may feel the use of first names early in the relationship is condescending. The therapist should know the meaning that first names have for clients before using them routinely.

The personalities of both therapist and client contribute to the outcome of the process. To understand and help clients, the therapist needs certain qualities (Carkhuff and Berenson, 1977; Rogers, 1957; Truax and Carkhuff, 1967). The kind of *person* the therapist is, regardless of theoretical orientation or technique, is the key to effective intervention. The therapist's humaneness, values, feelings, attitudes, and behavior all contribute greatly to the therapeutic relationship. Because communication involves mutual interaction, the client is in a position to perceive many of the therapist's true feelings. As Ellis (1955) states:

> The personality of the therapist is a most important factor in psychotherapy. . . . The therapist's deepest inner self, as well as his more external characteristics and manner, are, whether or not he is conscious of the fact, inevitably used in his therapeutic relationship; and it is by the use of himself as an instrument that he usually. . . helps effect significant changes in the self of the client.

Perhaps the next question is: How is the therapeutic relationship established? How is it brought about? In addition to being an able communicator, the therapist needs certain facilitative capacities: acceptance, respect, genuineness, nonjudgmental attitude, empathic understanding, and the capacity to elicit and to tolerate painful emotional feelings.

Acceptance. The basis of all therapeutic relationships is the acceptance of the client as a worthy and valuable person. Everyone needs to feel accepted throughout life. Acceptance means the individual has worth and value; that he or she deserves the therapist's time and efforts to help. Many persons do not seek help because they are afraid they will be considered unimportant. Others approach the setting anticipating rejection. Consequently the therapist must communicate a feeling of acceptance to the client, not verbally but affectively and behaviorally. The therapist does not have to take any specific action; he or she will communicate feelings verbally and nonverbally when the feelings are there.

The concept of acceptance should not be confused with blanket approval of all human behavior, especially dastardly acts such as rape, child abuse, assault, or homicide. But although the therapist dislikes those acts, he or she can still accept the individual as worthy of the effort to help. Generally, the therapist should be able to accept anyone for two reasons: (a) because the therapist has a need to help others, and (b) because the therapist understands human motivation and wants to understand the client. The therapist knows that all human behavior is motivated, purposeful, and is an individual effort to meet needs. The client with the worst behavior does not need condemnation from the therapist, but an effort at understanding so that the client can be helped to meet needs more constructively.

The client, no matter what he or she does, must feel accepted in order to feel worthy and to develop confidence in the therapist. The client must willingly express feelings and must be able to deal with problems and self safely, honestly, and effectively. As Biestek (1957) states: "The purpose of acceptance is therapeutic; to aid . . . in understanding the client as he really is."

It should be clear that acceptance cannot take place unless the therapist is sincere and has respect for the dignity of all human beings. These feelings are a product of socialization and life experiences that accumulate before a person becomes a therapist; training, knowledge, and education only intensify them. If these feelings are not already there in the individual, all the knowledge, training, and education in the world will not make that individual an effective therapist.

Empathic Understanding. Another capacity instrumental to establishing a therapeutic relationship is empathic understanding, which is an extension of the process of empathy. Empathy occurs through identification; the therapist shares the feelings of the client by projecting himself or herself into the client's situation. Although this enables the therapist to feel what the client feels, the therapist still must maintain objectivity and control emotional involvement. It is a form of saying, "I know how you feel."

Empathy is often confused with sympathy. Feeling sympathy connotes feeling sorry for a person, not only for suffering but also because of the hopelessness of the condition or situation. Feeling sympathy does not mean sharing feelings. In empathy there are shared feelings, but there is also confidence or hope that something can be done to improve the situation. The therapist who has sympathy rather than empathy communicates a feeling of hopelessness to the client.

The crisis therapist must take empathy one step farther, to emphatic understanding. Empathic understanding means the therapist not only has empathy but has the capacity to communicate it to the client. Again, the therapist does not have to demonstrate empathic understanding directly or dramatically; it will be communicated if it is there. The client will know when he or she is understood and feelings are shared. Again, the therapist's sincerity and respect for the client are important. Empathic understanding cannot be artificial. If the therapist says, "I understand," it must be at a time when he or she actually feels that way and also feels that the client needs to be reassured. It should never be said simply because it is "good technique."

Sometimes a client will ask the therapist, "Do you understand me?" This is important because of its possible meanings. It could mean the client feels the therapist is not communicating understanding effectively. Or if the client is accustomed to being misunderstood, he or she may just assume that the therapist does not understand. If the therapist does understand, the client's question should be briefly explored. For example, it might be beneficial for the therapist to say, "I think I understand you quite well. Is there something about me that makes you think that I don't understand you?" The client's responses give the therapist information about the client's perceptions and whether something he or she is not aware of is being communicated. In addition, they help the client become aware of the interaction in the relationship and of differences in perception.

Acceptance of Painful Feelings. A third important characteristic is the therapist's ability to elicit and tolerate painful feelings, regardless of content. A crisis, by definition, is an extremely painful emotional state, one that people try desperately to avoid. But for the person in crisis, avoiding the painful feelings is harmful. Consequently the therapist must be able to help the client face these feelings with responses that encourage their maximum expression, regardless of what or how painful the feelings are. The therapist too, must be able to tolerate such pain. Helping the client face painful emotional feelings not only facilitates the therapist's understanding of the client's condition, but it strengthens the client's ego because the client has the therapist's support in facing feelings that were faced alone before. If the therapist has difficulty tolerating painful affect, he or she might try to make the client feel better before the client has sufficiently expressed his or her emotional feelings.

The capacity of a therapist to establish a therapeutic relationship depends on the kind of person the therapist is. It depends on the capacity to accept people as they are, to be honest and sincere. It depends on the capacity to communicate empathic understanding and on the ability to elicit and tolerate the client's painful emotions.

Quite frequently, warmth is associated with a therapeutic relationship. But again, the therapist should not act artificially warm. An expression of warmth should be the intrinsic feelings of the therapist brought out by the client's need for help. The therapist should not strive to be warm but simply to be natural and not to be oversolicitous. Perhaps the client wants above all to be accepted and understood. This should be the consequence of a natural human relationship, nothing artificial or contrived. One of the most important factors in therapeutic success is knowing when and how to communicate respect, empathy, and understanding.

The techniques of interviewing that facilitate the therapeutic relationship can now be discussed.

TECHNIQUES OF INTERVIEWING

Techniques of interviewing are separated from the techniques of intervention to emphasize the information gathering phase of the treatment process.

Although the word "technique" has a connotation of a mechanical or manipulative approach, it is a precise explanation of what the therapist does. For the purpose of this book, the word *technique* is used to identify the skill portion of the therapeutic process—the manner of performance. Techniques are what the therapist does to make things happen and to achieve the therapeutic goal. The three major techniques of therapeutic interviewing are observing, listening, and questioning and exploring.

Observing

It may seem strange to consider observation a technique of interviewing. Nevertheless it is, and it requires a great deal of skill. Observation is a technique used from the beginning of the therapeutic process until the process is terminated. The therapist uses knowledge of human behavior and consciously observes the client to collect information. The first use of the technique of observation is noting the nonverbal signs sent by the client in the preinterview stage. These are the therapist's first clues to understanding the client. What does the therapist observe about the client? First, the therapist observed the client's dress and physical appearance. Although there is a great deal of freedom today in choice of dress and personal appearance, they still can be significant. Dress and personal appearance are forms of self-expression. They can reflect an individual's state of mind, body image, self-concept, or membership in a certain cultural subgroup. However, the significance of dress and personal appearance for the crisis therapist is how they reflect the client's condition. Dress is generally consistent with position in life—with age, sex, occupation, culture and socioeconomic status. If the dress and personal appearance of the person in crisis vary significantly from expected patterns, they most often reflect the crisis condition. They may indicate lowered self-esteem, and a decreased interest in self and personal relationships. On the other hand, the person in crisis who continues to maintain his or her customary dress and personal appearance may show a higher level of ego functioning, of hope, and motivation for help. Concern with maintaining customary patterns of dress and personal appearance indicates the individual's desire to maintain human contact and personal relationships, which are vital needs for the person in crisis.

The importance of the observation of physical appearance is twofold: it can indicate (a) how an individual takes care of himself or herself or (b) whether there is bodily abuse through drugs, alcohol, or inadequate diet.

Second, the therapist observes the client's gait, posture, gestures, nonverbal facial expressions, and affect. These will also be observed during the interview, but the therapist should be sensitive to them from the first time the client is seen. Gait and posture are fairly easy to interpret. A slow methodical gait can show depression, fatigue, discouragement, or lack of interest, for example. On the other hand, a rapid gait could represent anxiety, fear, or agitation. Posture, like gait, very often expresses a specific mood or affect, from the person who slumps in a chair to one who perches on the edge of the seat. Also, posture may reflect changes in affect during the course of the interview. An example is the client who rocks continuously in the chair until the therapist says something significant, and suddenly stops rocking. Posture can also indicate boredom and lack of interest.

Most gestures are hand movements. They can show anger or emphasis (e.g., clenching a fist, pointing a finger, or pounding on the table).

They can represent anxiety and depression (e.g., nailbiting, wringing the hands, chain-smoking). The hands can express feelings of confusion, discouragement, or hopelessness. Perhaps the most accurate nonverbal expressions of true feelings are facial expressions, including the eyes. Facial expressions reflect certain feelings; they mirror joy, sadness, pain, approval or disapproval, interest of lack of interest, enthusiasm, boredom, anxiety, depression. The eyes also can reflect hope or sadness. They can reflect shyness or low self-esteem. And they reflect feelings about others as well as self. The way one person looks at another can express love, hate, or curiosity. The individual who is unable to look at another may be indicating shyness or dishonesty. At other times, the eyes may reflect mistrust or a desire for privacy. Wearing sunglasses during the interview can mean that the client is trying to hide distress or does not want anyone to know where he or she is looking. Or it could mean only that the person is shy. But the wearing of sunglasses is almost always significant; it certainly prevents eye contact.

In the interview situation, facial expressions and affect occur simultaneously with verbal expressions. Generally, they are used to support, emphasize, or reinforce verbal messages. However, many times there is a discrepancy between verbal communication and facial expressions and affect. When there is a difference between nonverbal and verbal expressions, the former are most often a more accurate reflection of true feelings than the latter. This is because most nonverbal messages are not consciously sent, and the individual is not really aware of their meaning. The most accurate communication of feelings occurs when verbal communication and nonverbal communication reflect the same basic meaning. If a person says he or she is angry, nonverbal communication should reflect this anger. If a person says he or she is angry but smiles or does not look or act angry, that person either is not angry or is greatly suppressing angry feelings.; The appropriate expression of feelings, both verbally and nonverbally, is especially important for the person in crisis. Consequently, not only should there be careful observation of inconsistent verbal and nonverbal messages, but also of inappropriate communication. That is, the therapist should observe whether the client is expressing appropriate feelings that are consistent with the precipitating event. If not, the real feelings may be going on internally. When this occurs the therapist should usually bring it to the client's attention. For example, the therapist might say, "You seem to be talking about something that is very distressing to you, but you don't look as if it bothers you as much as I would expect."

Observation is a very important technique involving constant attention to all of the client's behavior, interpreting its meaning, and using it to help the client. This will become clearer when all of the techniques of interviewing are discussed, since the process is a unified whole.

Listening

A second important interviewing technique is listening. Listening well is more complicated and requires more than you might think. It requires the therapist's full attention to be alert, observant, and sensitive to the meaning of words and language. Therapeutic listening requires the therapist to put aside personal thoughts and to keep the mind from wandering. It requires a genuine and intense interest in the client.

It is very important that the therapist not take the client's communication for granted, and not assume that he or she knows what the client means. The therapist cannot assume what the client means simply because a common word is used; that assumption can lead to misunderstanding. Recall that many factors affect the communication process, including a lifetime of experiences. Self-concept, preservation of self-image, educational level, image of the therapist, status relationship, and expectation also influence the way a person communicates. Since each word has a unique meaning associated with the individual's personal experiences, the assumption that they have the same meaning for the client and the therapist is subject to error. The therapist should try to understand what the client is saying from the client's psychic reality. The therapist must feel free to ask the client what is meant or let the client know he or she does not understand if a client is using an ambiguous word. Even when the therapist is reasonably sure what the client means, the therapist should question it if the client seems unsure or vague. Such questioning helps the client to focus, to identify problems, and put them in clearer perspective. The basis of questioning is listening.

Like observation, listening is a technique for gathering data about the client. It involves hearing what the client is saying literally and understanding what the client means. To understand completely, the therapist must be attentive and concentrate on what the client is saying. The therapist must understand the meaning of words, language, affect, and nonverbal communication. The therapist must be sensitive to emotionally laden words and should have a clear picture of the client's problems and conflicts and the reasons they exist.

Listening begins with the client's opening statement, and the therapist should pay special attention to it. Some clients start discussing problems right away; others fill the first minutes of the interview with social amenities. Still others start with an expression of doubt or hopelessness: "I don't know whether you can help me, but . . ." or "I don't think anything can be done, but . . ." Sometimes these statements are requests for encouragement or for brief reassurance that the therapist can help or is willing to. At other times the client expresses concerns forthrightly and requires no response from the therapist.

Regardless of what the client's opening statement is, special consideration should be given to what is being communicated and how and why it is being communicated. The opening statement sometimes (but not always) establishes what is most important to the client. This initial interaction between client and therapist can determine the success or failure of the interview. Sullivan (1954) calls this the *formal inception* stage.

Once the interview is past the opening phase, the therapist's goal is to understand the client as thoroughly as possible. The therapist first listens to the meaning of each sentence, being careful to hear all emotionally laden words that reflect either the client's feelings about what he or she is saying or a concern that is not being communicated directly. To further understand what the client is saying, the therapist must consider the sum of all sentences over a period of time. The meaning of each sentence is determined by the ones that preceded it.

The therapist should be able to determine the client's basic concern, which may not always be what is verbalized. For example, Larry was highly distressed on hearing of the illness of his best friend's father. But his distress was not so much out of concern for the sick person but out of worry for himself. He tends to overidentify with illness and accidents because of his preoccupation with himself. His worry about his friend's father seemed very altruistic but actually had other significance.

The therapist must listen not only to what the client talks about but also to what the client avoids talking about. For instance, the married client who does not eventually discuss the marital relationship is probably not facing something of significance.

In addition, the therapist should pay strict attention to the client's nonverbal messages. He or she should listen to changes in tone of voice or in rate of speech. The therapist should note the topics covered and the circumstances of each change. Such changes can indicate a change in feelings or a desire to avoid the pain associated with some topic. It is also significant when the client mentions a subject more than once or repeatedly returns to the same subject. This could mean that the topic is so important to the client that he or she is preoccupied with it and cannot move on. The client may be trying to resolve a painful subject by facing it repeatedly, the way the soldier returns to fight a lost battle. Another possible meaning is that the pain associated with the subject matter is so great that the client needs to repeat it because he or she is hurt and disappointed. This is really a form of disbelief or denial. A client may repeat a topic because he or she feels that the therapist is not hearing the message; the client may repeat it until the therapist hears and responds in a way the client finds appropriate.

It is very important for the therapist to understand the sequence of the client's messages. If the client is coherent, the facts should be reasonably interrelated. However, this is not always the case with people in crisis, especially when they are emotionally upset. The therapist must notice when the client's communication is not clear or is inconsistent. At this time questions designed to help the therapist understand will also help the client to think more logically and to gain a better perspective on his or her condition. By the completion of the first interview, there should be very few, if any, questions about the client that the therapist cannot answer.

Questioning and Exploring

Questioning and exploring are techniques used to elicit responses and to help clients talk freely and constructively. They are often used together. In fact, questions are used in exploring.

Questioning has several purposes in therapeutic work: (a) to gather data; (b) to understand the client's condition; (c) to motivate the client to pursue a specific topic or subject matter; and (d) to help the client clarify thoughts. Questioning helps clarify the client's confusion and reestablish logic.

Exploring means delving into a topic in depth. It lets the therapist and client share the client's experiences for as long as the client is willing. It can be used to help the client express powerful feelings essential in resolving the crisis.

Exploration requires the therapist to tolerate painful emotions. It means getting the client to share feelings, regardless of how painful the feelings are. It may even mean getting the client to face his or her own death or the death of a loved one. As Brill (1978) says in the preface to her book:

> Soon after the first edition of this book was published, a woman came to see me and asked if I would help her to live till she died and to die with dignity. She had just learned that she had advanced cancer of the pancreas and her time was short. We met once or twice a month, had lunch together, talked, shared readings, ideas, and feelings. She worked as long as she was able, participated in seminars on dying and death, shared her life with her family and friends, died as she had wished.

Success in exploration requires the utmost skill. It should not be confused with probing, a questioning technique without the affective component used to gain information. The purpose of exploration is to encourage the sharing and expression of feelings as well as to gain information.

Two different skills are involved in questioning and exploring: timing and formulating. Timing is the ability to know when to ask a question without interfering with the flow of the client's conversation. A question appropriately timed is not an interruption or obstacle to the client's communication but encourages the client to elaborate on what he or she is saying, to discuss additional feelings and ideas, to continue talking. The therapist should always stay where the client is, and ask questions only at the time that the topic is either on the client's mind or in the conversation. Questioning should not be used to change the subject unless the client has completely exhausted the subject matter. And even though the therapist may need specific information to assess the client, the client always provides clues for a smooth transition from subject to subject. The therapist should skillfully guide the client when necessary by logically sequencing questions based on what the client is saying. For example, a client may say, "I've been throwing away a lot of old junk and some of my good books that I'm tired of reading." The therapist knows that, quite often, throwing or giving away valuable possessions can be a clue to suicide ideation. Although the client's statement appears almost trivial, the fact that the client even mentions it to the therapist makes it significant. In spite of apparent insignificance, the therapist should use such messages as signals; in this case, to explore suicidal thoughts. The therapist might ask the client about the client's motivation for throwing away the books, and then ask if he had thought about taking his own life.

Appropriately timed questions give the client the impression that many subjects have been covered but that there has been one continuous interview. If the therapist follows the principle of staying where the client is and always having a purpose for questions, they will almost always be appropriate and relevant.

The second skill in questioning and exploring is formulating, or phrasing. Because the therapist is most interested in the client's expression of feelings and ideas, most questions should be designed to encourage the client to express feelings openly and freely. Thus the crisis therapist's questions should be open ended. That is, they should require explanations and discussion rather than yes-or-no answers. The therapist's questions should start with what, how, when, or where, not with why. Questions beginning with why require a cognitive answer: they may make the client feel defensive and as if he or she is being examined. Furthermore, it is easy to answer, "I don't know" to a why question. Why questions remind people of childhood and of parents and teachers. They carry blame and accusation. Questions such as, "What brought that about?" "How did that happen?" "What do you think are some possible reasons for your reactions?" "What does that mean to you?" "What happened to make you want to leave?" are more likely to evoke honest, undefensive reactions. Such questions lead people to explore their feelings—to be introspective. For example, if the therapist asks a client, "How are things going?" the client will generally respond with whatever is important to him or her. If the therapist asks a closed question, the client will give a specific answer that may not be very important at the time. Furthermore, the therapist's questions should not be "loaded": they should not require the client to admit to something negative, as would a question such as "Don't you think that ignoring your wife's birthday makes her angry?" A more effective way to phrase the question would be, "What is the effect of ignoring your wife's birthday?" In therapeutic interviewing, the goal is to discover feelings as well as facts; open questions are thus more useful. The therapist should not use leading questions that suggest a "right" answer.

Another part of successful questioning is the nonverbal component. Tone of voice is extremely important in determining how a question is received. A good, open-ended question designed to elicit discussion and the expression of feelings may be ruined if tone of voice and other nonverbal signals imply that there is a right answer or that certain answers might be condemned. As we discussed, if the therapist's face, tone of voice, or other nonverbal messages are not consistent with verbal expression, the client will usually respond to the nonverbal message. In addition, the language and vocabulary used should fit the client's educational level and frame of reference.

Thus far the discussion has focused on direct methods of questioning. There are also indirect methods such as reflection or restatement. To reflect or restate, the therapist repeats in a questioning tone an emotional word or sentence used by the client. Reflection and restatement are used when the therapist wants the client to hear what he himself (the client) is saying. They can be used to encourage the client to go into more detail on a subject.

Another indirect method is to form a question as a statement, such as, "That sounds really painful" or "That must have been really hard on you." This kind of questioning is used to get the client to share more feelings. It is used when a client may be a little reserved or reluctant to express painful feelings.

A third indirect method is the use of comparative questions. For example, to the wife who says her husband does not love her, the therapist could say, "By 'love' do you mean affection, or concern for your welfare?" The question stimulates the client to think about what love is and about whether there are some positive things in the relationship. The direct question, "What do you mean by 'love'?" could make the client defensive and reactivate basic feelings of being unloved.

There are times the therapist has to ask direct questions, most often to get factual information and demographic data. But even then, each question should be based on the previous discussion. The advice of Bernstein and Bernstein (1974) on formulating direct questions is useful. They state that: (a) the sequence of questions should progress from the general to the specific, (b) the questions should progress from the less personal to the more personal, (c) the questions should be worded to elicit answers of a sentence or more and to avoid yes and no responses, (d) the questions should be worded to avoid bias.

TECHNIQUES OF INTERVENTION

Intervention techniques are the methods used purposefully by a therapist to change or influence an individual's emotional or mental state or behavior. The distinction between interviewing and intervening is rather artificial; in practice they overlap and are parts of the same process. But we will distinguish between them on the basis of purpose. Interviewing facilitates the client's expression of feelings and awareness of experiences. It is done to let the therapist get to know the client as an individual and to gather information.

Intervention can have one of four basic purposes: (a) to restore the client's social functioning to a previous level, (b) to sustain a certain level of social functioning, (c) to improve the client's social functioning, or (d) to change various aspects of personality. Sometimes more than one of these goals is appropriate for the same client. However, the basic goal of *crisis intervention* is to restore the client's social functioning at least to the level at which the client was prior to the onset of the crisis.

We can divide the techniques of intervention into three categories: (a) psychological support, those techniques designed to sustain and support positive aspects of social functioning; (b) cognitive restoration, those designed to alter, change, or modify social functioning; and (c) environmental modification, those that change the relationship between the client and his or her environment. The crisis therapist may use all of these techniques with the same client.

Psychological Support

Every therapist uses support in some fashion. In fact, the therapeutic relationship is by nature a framework of support. Psychological support helps the client face problems that previously were faced alone. The overwhelming feelings produced by a crisis weaken the client's ability to function; he or she needs ego strength to master the crisis.

When the client needs support beyond what comes from a therapeutic relationship, it must be purposefully and skillfully given. The effective use of psychological support requires an understanding of the individual's personality. Giving support does not mean simply giving praise or saying common words of encouragement such as "You did a good job" or "You're a good person." Supportive words should go beyond maintaining the client's self-esteem; they should reinforce, sustain, or encourage positive or constructive feelings and behaviors. Supportive techniques are used to maintain the client's level of ego functioning or to motivate the client to try harder. They provide hope and develop confidence.

The basic skill involved in the use of support is timing. To know the most effective time to use support, the therapist must understand the individual's personality and decide when the client needs support and will effectively receive it. Not everyone wants to be praised or encouraged—not even all those in crisis. If the client feels guilty or inferior and self-esteem is low, supportive techniques might be ineffective. Even though the client may like to hear words of encouragement, he or she may not be ready to truly believe them. This is especially true for the depressed client. Remember that people who are depressed tend to turn inward or withdraw. During this time an internal battle is going on, and the client is suffering. For example, a grieving woman who is feeling guilty about her anger toward her dead mother may not want to hear that "everyone feels that he should have treated a lost loved one better." In such a situation, the therapist should listen until the client is ready for active intervention. Often, hearing positive support before the client is ready may increase guilt feelings. Other examples of people who cannot accept positive support include the strikingly beautiful woman or handsome man who feels unattractive. They do not feel beautiful on the inside. They may feel they cannot live up to the expectations of the people around them. A similar example is the very talented individual who feels undeserving despite achievements and accomplishments. These examples illustrate that the way people feel about themselves is more important to themselves than how others see or feel about them. And this self-image does not yield easily to popularity or premature compliments.

Of course, sometimes a depressed client will actively seek praise and reassurance at the same time the internal battle of self-blame and guilt is going on. The client may want to counteract the internal struggles with external praise. But while praise makes the client feel good for a short time, the good feelings generally do not last. Sometimes a client needs to experience painful emotions for a while before he or she can receive active psychological support. This does not mean the client is not being supported at all, but that he or she is not being *falsely* supported. The therapist can refrain from actively praising and supporting the client until psychological needs are understood.

The premature use of support presents other potential problems. It can make the client feel that the therapist does not consider the condition serious or that the condition is being taken too lightly. The client may feel that the therapist underestimates the difficulty of the problem. Premature support may cause the client to feel additional pressure to please the therapist or to be successful too soon.

Clients feeling anxious may be ready for more active support earlier than those experiencing depression. The person who is experiencing anxiety is outwardly directed and actively seeks help from others. The anxious client is more receptive to the direct action of the therapist than is the depressed client. In both cases, however, the use of active support should be purposeful and based on an understanding of the basic personality and needs of the client.

The most effective support comes from the therapeutic relationship and from within the client. Support is always more effective when the client shows readiness to receive the therapist's active support. The client will usually show signs of being ready by communicating it nonverbally, with eyes or facial expressions. It is often a good idea to check out the client's feelings about the need for support. Rather than reassure a client that he or she can do something, the therapist can first ascertain the client's feelings about whether he or she can do it. Instead of initially saying, "I think you can manage now," it may be more effective to say, "I wonder if you can manage now." The client's response can be followed with a test of conviction, such as "What makes you feel you *can* manage now?" This interaction communicates a shared responsibility for the client's social functioning. At the same time, the therapist has other evidence to evaluate the client's condition. Even in situations where the client's behavior is obviously constructive, his or her feelings about the behavior should be ascertained first. The active use of support should be based on three conditions. First, the therapist supports only constructive or positive feelings and behavior of the client. (Feelings and behavior that should not be supported can still be accepted; support means the therapist wants the behavior to continue; acceptance means that the therapist is able to value and respect the dignity of the individual, regardless of the behavior.) Second, the client communicates the need to be actively supported and that he or she will be receptive to it. Third, the therapist has already activated any self-support in the client.

Listening. Although listening is a technique of interviewing, it also can be used as a supportive technique. When used as a form of support, the therapist deliberately suspends response to the client and listens attentively to the client. Often, if the client talks freely to an interested therapist, he or she can arrive at an understanding of the condition and, very often, his or her own solution. When the therapist purposefully refrains from speaking, the client can gain strength from talking. The client is forced to rely on what he or she says and hears. Even if the client asks the therapist for a response, the therapist can say something like, "To really get the feel of what you're saying, I'd like you to talk a little longer before I answer your question." Often the client lets the therapist know when simple listening is needed. Nonverbal signals will say, "I want you just to listen." Research shows that the more the client talks and the less the therapist talks, the greater the chance of therapeutic success (Carnes and Robinson, 1948). The therapist's success is not determined by *how much* is said but by *what* is said.

Ventilation. One of the most useful techniques for the crisis therapist is ventilation, which involves eliciting powerful emotions so the client can experience those feelings and eventually master them. Ventilation involves exploration. For example, a therapist could say, "I can see that your relationship with your husband was truly important to you. I wonder if you can describe to me exactly how you feel now that he is gone." This type of explorative question not only draws out potent feelings but also helps the client face the reality of the situation by not pretending that her husband may come back. The use of ventilation must be done with empathy and, again, must be properly timed. It must not be done simply for the sake of technique.

Reassurance. Reassurance is a method by which the therapist conveys to the client that he or she can be helped, that the condition is not hopeless, that the perceived danger can be managed and resolved successfully, and that the client has more ability or greater strength than he or she may realize. Like all supportive techniques, reassurance should be used only when justified by the therapist's confidence in the truth of the client's statements. The therapist has to anticipate the future, based on both the client's past and the evidence presented at the time. If there is no basis for the therapist's reassurance, it is false and misleading. As with other techniques, reassurance should be used only after the client's need for it has been determined. The client's fears or lack of confidence should be directly expressed before the therapist gives reassurance. The client should respond to questions such as, "What makes you feel so pessimistic?" or "What makes you feel you can't do it?" before the therapist gives reassurance. The client may be seeking encouragement before taking action by asking, "Do you think I can find a new job?" If the therapist knows that the client thinks he or she has the ability but just wants to be reassured, the therapist can say something like, "I think you can find a job, and your past record suggests you can." If, on the other hand, the client feels pessimistic and hopeless, the therapist should not give reassurance but should express acceptance. He might say, "If you truly feel you cannot find a job and are afraid to try, we'll have to wait until you're ready." The therapist has to determine the client's readiness for the reassurance.

Reassurance can be used to help the client recognize abilities of which the client is unaware. It can also be used to help the client develop more trust and confidence in the therapist. For example, once the therapist has determined that the client needs reassurance and can be helped, he can say, "By working together I think we can be successful in resolving this problem." This kind of reassurance is often required in crisis therapy. Again, it cannot be falsely used. If a man is in crisis because his wife has unilaterally decided to get a divorce, reassurance that things can be worked out is not justified. Reassurance should never be used in a situation that is uncertain or hopeless. It should also never be used to allow the client to avoid taking responsibility for behavior or for facing the reality of the situation. Reassurance should be used to motivate the client and to help toward continued improvement.

Clarification. Clarification is a technique of support as well as of interviewing. It is used in interviewing to help the therapist understand the client and the situation. When used as a supportive technique, it causes the client to focus on a problem or to recognize that something is inconsistent or missing in what he or she is saying. It may also indicate that what the client is saying is so important the therapist wants the client to explore it further. Clarification helps the client expand perceptions. It often helps a client face a problem or a feeling he or she may want to avoid. Clarification should not be confused with interpretation. Clarification is concerned with the meaning of manifest feelings and behavior; interpretation is concerned with unconscious or latent feelings.

Clarification is also used when the therapist asks the client to clarify the meaning of what the client is saying. For example, the therapist might say, "Would you explain the difference between your feelings at the time of your husband's death and your father's?" Clarification can be used to reinforce a significant thought or feeling. For example, a therapist could say, "If I understand you correctly, you never had headaches before your mother-in-law came to live with you." There may not really have been anything unclear about the client's statement, but for clarity and reinforcement the therapist repeats the cause-and-effect relationship.

In addition, clarification can be used to elicit new material. For example, a therapist might say, "The relationship between your headaches and your mother-in-law is not clear to me." The client's response may lead to a discussion of his relationship with his wife. Perhaps he would say, "When my mother-in-law is in our home, my wife acts differently toward me." This response then opens other areas of concern.

Universalization. Universalization involves telling the client that the experience is a common human one and that the client's reaction is not unusual. It must be used with a clear understanding of its purpose and the client's receptivity to it. While there is strength in commonness, most people also need to be considered unique. However, when it is indicated, universalization can be quite effective. It can be reassuring to hear the therapist say, "It's natural for you to feel the way you do," or "If you didn't get angry at that, I'd be worried." Universalization is used *only* when the client is in a common situation and the reaction is typical. It is used only when the client needs reassurance that his or her feelings or behavior are common to all people.

Confrontation. Confrontation is used when the client resists facing the reality of the condition, feelings, or behavior. The client has to be confronted with this reluctance to face a feeling, behavior, or problem when failure to do so is counterproductive.

Confrontation directs the client toward facing something that he or she would rather not face. Thus it must be done supportively, without attacking. The therapist should move slowly at first; if the client responds to mild use of confrontation, more direct confronting may not be necessary. For example, the therapist may say, "For some reason you seem not to act on your dislike for your mother-in-law." In this case the therapist is confronting the client with the fact that, although he dislikes his mother-in-law, he is not doing anything about the situation except complaining. If this nonthreatening exchange stimulates the client to take action, no further confrontation is necessary. But if after a reasonable period of time no change occurs, a more direct confrontation may be indicated. For example, the therapist might say, "Knowing your feelings about your mother-in-law and the effect she has on you, perhaps it's time we look at what keeps you from doing something about it." If such a direct confrontation is not effective, then the therapist must look for other obstacles preventing the client from resolving the situation. In the above case, for example, perhaps the husband cannot do anything about the situation because he actually wants his mother-in-law's love and approval, but she will not respond to him the way he wants her to. Perhaps if he becomes aware of his real desires, confrontation will not be needed. An ineffective confrontation may mean the therapist has to set limits or take some direct action. For example, the therapist may say, "It looks like you can't come to grips with your feelings about your child. On this basis we must take active steps to help you and the child."

Persuasion. Persuasion is another method used to help the client overcome resistance to help. It is based on (a) the therapist's authority and the client's trust, and (b) the therapist's belief that the client will be successful if the therapist's wishes are carried out. Persuasion is used with people in crisis who are so debilitated by their situation they need a direct approach. Examples include persuading a teen-aged client to return home or a person with chest pains to go to the hospital. Even in such cases, persuasion should be used only after the therapist judges the client's own resources to be ineffective. For example, the therapist and the client should thoroughly discuss what the client thinks about returning home before the therapist tries to persuade him that going home is in his best interest. People who come to their own successful conclusions and make constructive decisions about their own lives are generally happier and stronger for it.

Suggestion. In effect, suggestion is a mild form of persuasion where the therapist is less insistent that the client do what the therapist says. With persuasion, the therapist is insistent and persistent. The use of both suggestion and persuasion should be based on the client's personality. Again, clients have greater self-respect when they arrive at their own solutions to problems; guiding clients to make the best use of their own resources is always the most effective intervention. Like persuasion, suggestion should be used only after other techniques have proved to be ineffective, even though people in crisis seem so helpless it is tempting to tell them what to do.

Advice. Advice involves the therapist telling someone—sometimes the client and sometimes a third party—what to do. In this context, advice means more than directive suggestion and persuasion. Its use should not be confused with recommending a course of action for a person in crisis. If a client has refused to respond to suggestion and persuasion and is endangering personal safety or that of others, the therapist may use advice. For example, the therapist might say, "It appears we can't work things out together. I advise you to immediately seek hospitalization." Or if a client refuses to go to the hospital, the therapist may advise the family to have the client admitted. Even then, all other alternatives should be exhausted before the therapist resorts to advice. It should be used only as a last resort.

Cognitive Restoration

The most salient characteristics of a person in crisis are overwhelming emotionality, confusion, and mental debilitation. An emotional crisis results in varying degrees of cognitive dysfunctioning. Therefore, one of the major goals of crisis intervention is the restoration of cognitive functioning. Before this can be done there must be some reduction in emotionality. The supportive techniques are designed to help reduce the client's emotionality; only then will the client be receptive to the techniques of cognitive restoration.

A considerable amount of client self-understanding results from interaction with the therapist and the process of interviewing. However, cognitive restoration is achieved by two therapeutic techniques: causal connecting statements and interpretation.

Causal Connecting Statement. A causal connecting statement is the process by which the therapist connects (or helps the client connect) the cause and effect of two events, conditions, or situations that have resulted in the client's specific feeling, behavior, or responses. It differs from interpretation in that explanations are based on the client's overt communication and expressions rather than on unconscious implications. The effect, a causal connecting statement, seeks to establish for the client a causal relationship between a series of events. Consider the following example:

Therapist: Hi! My name is Jack Stein. Can you tell me what brings you here?
Client: The nurse brought me here. I can't do my job. I feel like I'm falling apart.
Therapist: What do you mean by falling apart?
Client: This happened about a year ago. My girlfriend and I were having problems. I took my ring back because she did not do what I wanted her to, and then I tried to kill myself by cutting my wrist.
Therapist: (*causal connecting statement*) It sounds like when you feel like you are "falling apart" it means that you are in such great desperation and feel so hopeless that you think of suicide and attempt to take your own life.

It can be seen that a causal connecting statement ties together for the client the cause and effect of certain events and responses. Consider another example:

Client: I know it's not being a good mother to spank Chris every time he cusses at me. If I ignored it, he would soon stop. But I can't help myself.
Therapist: (*causal connecting statement*) In effect you are saying that Chris's cussing at you makes you feel you are a bad mother. Could it be possible that you are punishing Chris more for his making you feel like a bad mother than for his cussing?

It should be noted that causal connecting statements as well as interpretations are given with qualifications and tentativeness. This gives the client a chance to participate, to think over, to accept and integrate or to reject. If the client accepts and integrates, it becomes part of his or her cognitive functioning.

Interpretation. Interpretation is the second basic technique of cognitive restoration. Some experiential or affective learning takes place within the structure of the therapeutic relationship. However, interpretation is conscious and purposeful learning. In effect, everyone uses interpretation when offering an explanatory inference of the cause and meaning of some human behavior. When asking and answering why, an explanation is derived from certain data or evidence. This is interpretation. For the person in crisis, identifying what is happening emotionally and situationally is very important in resolving the problem. Interpretation helps the client think and perceive feelings and behavior from a more logical perspective. It restores order and structure to the individual's emotional life, which has been out of control. When the therapist identifies what is occurring within the client—some of which is unconscious—and why it is occurring, the client can understand the situation, which helps reduce the debilitating effect.

Interpretation is the crisis therapist's explanation of the cause and meaning of the client's feelings and behavior, to promote self-understanding and reestablishment of cognitive control. It gives the client an explanation of his or her behavior in the same way a physician gives a patient the meaning of physical symptoms. Interpretation involves making the client conscious of feelings and behavior of which he or she is unaware; it offers reasons and causes rather than describing what is already known. Interpretation involves relaying information to the client in tentative terms, or raising "think" questions regarding the cause, meaning, and purpose of unconscious behavior or feelings.

Hammer (1968) says that "other than the relationship-theory aspects (the patient feeling a sense of support, a relationship with someone who cares, a sense of trust) one of the first gains the patient generally struggles to acquire is being able to identify what is going on affectively and rationally." Fenichel (1945) states, "The verbalization of unclear worries alone brings relief because an ego can face verbalized ideas better than unclear emotional sensations." In crisis therapy, deep unconscious interpretation is unnecessary. What is necessary for cognitive restoration is the explanation of what is going on within the client, which enables the client to gain cognitive mastery over confusing and overwhelming affect. In this case, interpretation can take two forms: (a) informing the client of unconscious behavior involving current life situations (e.g., interpersonal relationships involving parents, spouse, and significant others) or conflicts in goals (e.g., self-defeating behavior), and (b) behavior that is a reflection of historical development and experiences involving specific patterns of psychic functioning. This is simply a matter of relating the past to the present. The basis of interpretation is knowledge and understanding of human behavior and a specific interest in helping the client understand his or her behavior.

Consider Scott, a social agency worker supporting a family, who wants to give up his job to enter private practice at considerable personal and financial risk. The therapist might say, "I wonder if your anger about not being able to enter private practice immediately is a result of your competition with me." This response might help Scott look at the meaning of his behavior in a new way. The following dialogue between Martha, a client who developed anxiety while in church, and her therapist is another example of interpretation:

Martha: While sitting in church, all of a sudden I felt faint and I experienced heavy feelings in my chest, began perspiring, and I had to leave the services. I felt better when I got outside.
Therapist: How do you explain this sudden attack of anxiety?
Martha: Well, I've been on a diet; and yesterday I ate a small piece of pie. It probably upset my sugar balance.

After exploring further, the therapist asked Martha what was going on at the time of her stress. She responded that the choir was singing about Christ's death and resurrection. Based on understanding of Martha, the therapist responded:

Therapist: Could it be that the words of the song stirred up some feelings of your own death, feelings that are frightening to you?
Martha: Well, this is Easter, and you know my father died of a heart attack last year at this time. I've always had a weak heart.

This particular interpretive question by the therapist gave Martha the clue to her own anxiety.

Another example of interpretation is, "Could it be that you ran away to test your parent's love for you and to express your anger at them by making them worry about you? Could that be possible?" The therapist's synthesis of the client's bewildering array of feelings helps the client organize thoughts. It facilitates the client's mastery of the condition and situation.

Interpretation should not be used until a good therapist-client relationship has been established. Even then it should be done in a supportive, nonthreatening manner. Use of interpretation is discussed further in Chapter 5.

Environmental Modification

The third technique of intervention is *environmental modification.* It means recommending either that the client be removed from a harmful environment or that the nature of the environment be changed.

Examples of removing a client from a harmful environment include the recommendation that a client be hospitalized or placed in a foster home. Changing the environment involves other people in the client's life. The therapist may need to work with a client's parents, spouse, or employer, with a financial agency, or with other social agencies. Environmental modification can be called for by three different conditions: (a) the client is not capable of improving as long as he or she remains in the current specific environment, (b) the client is not able to change the environment constructively, (c) environmental modification is needed as an adjunct to supportive intervention.

To use environmental modification the therapist must be familiar with community resources. Every crisis therapist should maintain an up-to-date file on all community resources, social agencies, and businesses and organizations that serve people.

Knowledge and skill in the use of techniques of interviewing and intervention facilitate helping people in crisis. In chapter 5 we will discuss the procedures of working with people in crisis.

SUMMARY

This chapter discussed the process and techniques of crisis intervention. The process begins when a significant event occurs in the life of an individual or family that cannot be resolved by the repeated efforts of usual coping and problem-solving methods. Progressively, some form of emotionalism becomes overwhelming, causing a crisis condition. The techniques of interviewing and intervention were discussed in the context of the therapeutic relationship.

REFERENCES

Bernstein, L., & Bernstein, R. (1974). *Interviewing: A guide for health professionals.* New York: Appleton-Century-Crofts.

Biestek, F. B. (1957). *The casework relationship.* Chicago: Loyola University Press.

Brill, N. I. (1978). *Working with people: The helping process.* Philadelphia: J. B. Lippincott.

Carkhuff, R. B., & Berenson, B. G. (1977). *Beyond counseling and therapy* (2nd ed.). New York: Holt, Rinehart and Winston.

Carnes, E. F., & Robinson, F. P. (1948). The role of client talk in the counseling interview. *Educational and Psychological Measurement, 8,* 635–644.

Ellis, A. (1955). New approaches to psychotherapy techniques. *Journal of Clinical Psychology, 11,* 208–260.

Fenichel, O. (1945). *The psychoanalytic theory of neurosis.* New York: W. W. Norton.

Hammer, E. F. (1968). *Use of interpretation in treatment: Technique and art.* New York: Grune & Stratton.

Rogers, C. R. (1957). Necessary and sufficient conditions of therapeutic personality change. *Journal of Consulting Psychology, 21,* 95–103.

Sullivan, H. S. (1954). *The psychiatric interview.* New York: W. W. Norton.

Truax, C. B., & Carkhuff, R. R. (1967). *Toward effective counseling and psychotherapy.* Chicago: Aldine.

Viney, L., Clarke, A. M., Bunn, T. A., & Benjamin, Y. M. (1985). Crisis intervention: An evaluation of long and short-term effects. *Journal of Counseling Psychology, 32*(1), 29–39.

SUGGESTED READINGS

Haley, J. (1976). *Problem solving therapy.* San Francisco: Jossey-Bass.

Hammer, E. F. (Ed.). (1968). *Use of interpretation in treatment: Technique and art.* New York: Grune & Stratton.

Kahn, R. L., & Cannell, C. F. (1957). *The dynamics of interviewing.* New York: John Wiley & Sons.

PART II

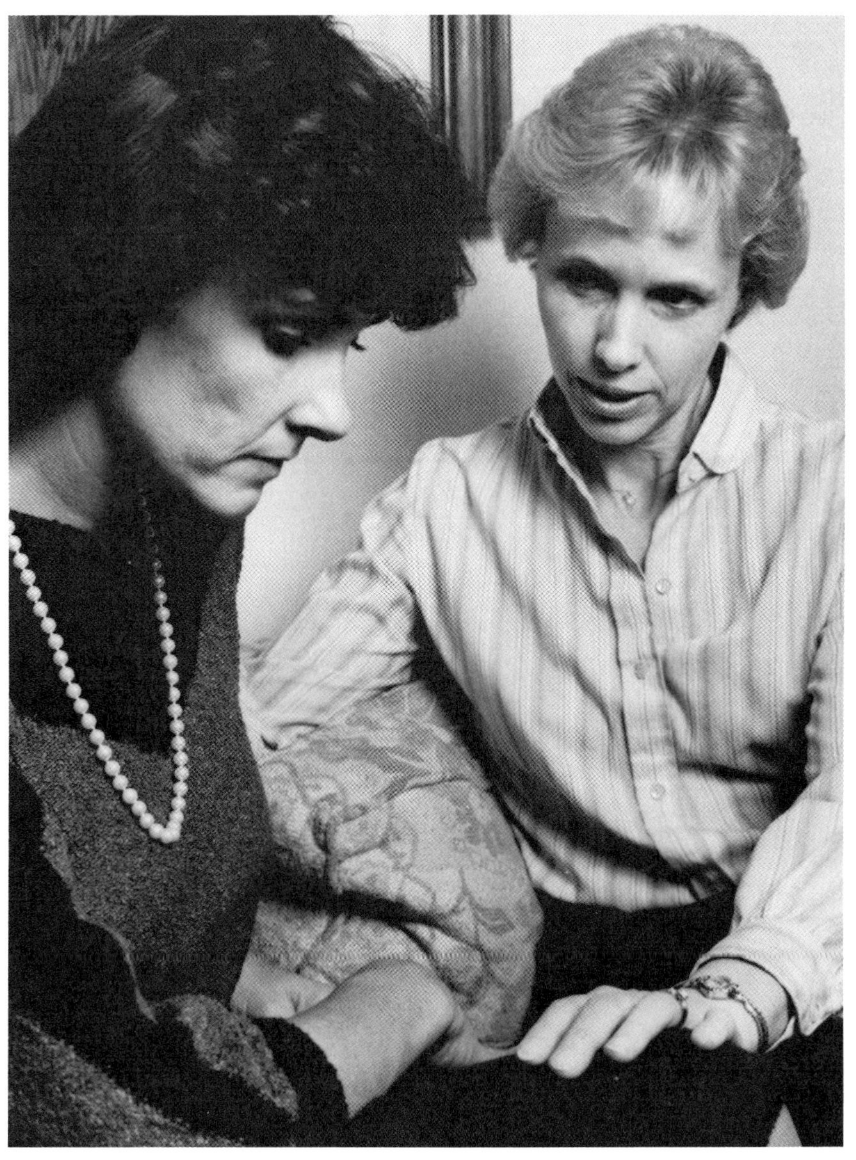

Application of Intervention Techniques and Skill Development

5

Procedures for Working with People in Crisis

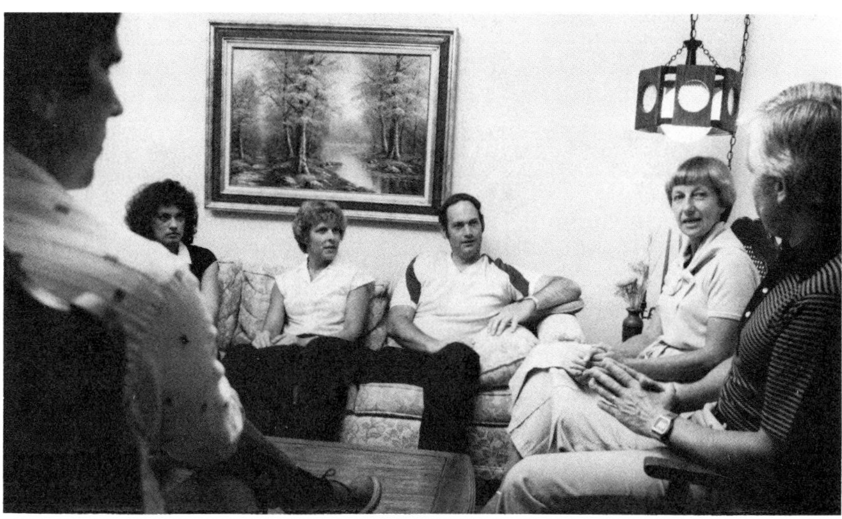

Case Studies

Mabel, age 41, was brought to the emergency service of the mental health clinic by her brother. He reported that Mabel had taken a large dose of Thorazine, a major tranquilizer, two hours earlier. The doctor who was consulted recommended she be kept in a protected environment for at least four more hours. He wanted to prevent Mabel from accidentally hurting herself. Mabel was obviously drug intoxicated. She was quite resistant to his recommendation because she had made plans to spend the evening with friends. Fortunately, a therapist was able to convince her to stay. Once she had decided to stay, Mabel fell asleep. On awaking several hours later, she decided that she had not had any intent to commit suicide, showed considerable improvement, and was eager to get home.

Forty-three-year-old Jane appeared at the crisis center depressed and seeking help. Some nine months earlier she had taken a job in a company she described as closed, negative, and debilitating. She had tried to change the system, but to no avail. She felt that leaving the situation would be like running away, and she had never run away from a battle in her life. She had lost weight and hated herself for being unable to do more to change the company.

Karen, 45 years old, reported to the crisis center complaining of difficulty eating and sleeping and with poor feelings about herself. She sleeps only one hour at night and one hour during the day. She can recognize her own considerable anger directed at herself, the source of which is conflict with family members. Although she currently is living with her sister, she wants out; she feels a need to be more independent. She also feels that her sister had changed since their uncle died and left the sister some money.

George, age 31, walked into the emergency service unit of the mental health clinic asking for help for his depression and the problems he was having with his girlfriend. He felt so depressed he was afraid he might do something "silly."

The former lover of 24-year-old Phyllis called the Crisis Center to refer her because he was worried about her. He had recently broken off their extramarital affair. She was now so depressed he feared she might take her own life. The therapist spoke with Phyllis, who at the time was crying but said she did not know why she was upset. She was given an immediate appointment.

These are samples of calls to emergency services and crisis units. You can see that when a person is in crisis, there is considerable confusion. The problems and causes are vague and often ill-defined. You can also see the wide variety of problems that can lead to a crisis, and the wide variety of reactions to those problems. The crisis therapist needs far-reaching knowledge to be able to work effectively with people in crisis. The first four chapters of this book focused on the theory of crisis, human behavior, communication, and the techniques used to improve, sustain, and alter social functioning. The remainder of the book will focus on using this knowledge in practice as we set forth procedural steps for effective intervention.

BASIC ATTITUDE AND APPROACH

Working with people in crisis requires a different attitude and approach than does traditional therapy. The crisis therapist must be willing and able to see the person in crisis as soon as possible. This is crucial; the client in crisis is most amenable to help at the time of the request for help and at the peak of the crisis. At this time the events precipitating the crisis are most accessible. The individual is less defensive and generally more introspective. In addition, immediately seeing the person in crisis reduces the chance that maladaptive efforts to resolve the crisis will become crystalized and the chance that compromise benefits of secondary gains will be acquired (Kalis, Harris, Prestwood, and Freeman, 1961).

In addition, consider Ben (see chapter 2), whose crisis was precipitated by his wife leaving him after he had beaten her. At the peak of his crisis he called a local agency, which offered him an appointment three days later. During those three days he attempted suicide and had to be hospitalized. Since the crisis was not resolved but the threat of suicide was abated, the psychiatrist at the hospital referred Ben back to the same agency. This case shows the importance of knowing when a person is in crisis. A crisis is subjectively defined by the individual; that is, initially a person is in crisis when he believes that he is in crisis, feels that he is unable to function, and turns to someone else for help. At this point some assessment and evaluation are needed, even if over the telephone. If the therapist cannot see the client immediately, the client should be referred to someone who can. In Ben's case, the therapist who spoke with him should have made some effort to evaluate him rather than routinely giving him the next available appointment. If the therapist could not see Ben, referral to another agency with some assurance that he got there was in order. What if Ben's interim suicide attempt had been successful? Most important, the case of Ben illustrates the need for staff and agencies to have a structure that allows people in crisis to be seen immediately. In fact, this should be a part of any helping agency, because people in crisis may call an agency other than a crisis center. They often call agencies whose names and services are familiar to them.

Of course, there are people who believe everything is a crisis and want to be seen every time they are upset. Most often these people are overly dependent on the agency and have not learned from previous crisis experiences. Assessment and evaluation and knowledge of these clients, too, are needed for appropriate responses. It seems important to evaluate why they are not becoming more independent and functioning better. The therapist needs to determine the meaning of the client's behavior. What prevents the client from making progress? People who are always in a crisis state are possible candidates for long-term psychotherapy. When this is not possible, the crisis model will probably have to suffice.

Another necessary approach is early assessment and evaluation of whether the individual needs hospitalization or can be helped on an outpatient basis. This is a question that concerns many crisis therapists, especially novices. From the first contact with the client through termination, the crisis therapist must keep this question in mind.

The crisis therapist *must* be self-confident. The multitude of problems presented by people in crisis can be very frightening as well as taxing. We have already seen the significance of confidence to client improvement. Anxiety and lack of confidence tend to be contagious. The opposite is also true: a calm, confident, hopeful therapist is very reassuring to a person in crisis.

PREPARATION FOR INTERVENTION

As previously stated, the first four chapters of this book have provided the conceptual and theoretical knowledge necessary to work with people in crisis. This chapter and those that follow apply that knowledge to the practice of crisis intervention.

Thinking Theoretically

It is generally agreed that crisis theory draws on several theories of human behavior, including ego psychology, system theory, learning theory, and humanism. It is less important whether a crisis therapist adheres to a particular theory or is eclectic as long as the therapist has a systematic basis for understanding, explaining, and evaluating human behavior. Functionally, a theory is a model of some aspect of reality; in this case, it is a model of human behavior. Thinking theoretically, then, is the application of a theoretical model to observed behavior as the client reveals problems, feelings, thoughts, and behavior.

To illustrate this process, let us draw upon an abbreviated version of ego psychology (Hartmann, 1958, Erikson, 1959, 1963). In ego psychology, emotional, psychological and cognitive functions are assigned to the three parts of the psychic system: ego, superego, and id. A person's memory, perception, thinking patterns, and judgment are considered ego functions. Conscience, self-evaluation, and self-esteem are considered superego functions. Inner stimuli for human behavior such as instincts, drives, needs, and feelings are considered id functions (although some needs also exist in the ego). Human behavior or psychosocial functioning is understood to be the qualitative, interrelated functioning of the three parts of the psychic system in the context of the social environment. The individual and the social environment are an interrelated, inseparable unit that must be considered in the total evaluation. To assess psychosocial functioning, the therapist observes how the ego, the superego, and the id are fulfilling their respective functions in the face of the crisis in the client's particular social environment.

Thinking theoretically, the crisis therapist empathizes and listens to the client, cognitively relating the client's feelings, expressions, actions, and behavior to the appropriate theoretical concept. For example, if the client states, "I feel guilty and ashamed," the therapist identifies that expression as conscience (superego function). If the client states, "I was unable to decide between going on vacation with my wife and her parents, or staying at home and suffering the consequences," the therapist thinks, what conflict caused this (indecisive functioning of the ego)? Guided by theoretical concepts, intervention at this point takes the form of questioning, clarifying, and encouraging as the therapist relates the client's feelings, verbal expressions, and behavior to the theoretical concept they reflect. The goal is to achieve total understanding, which does not mean to assume understanding, but to ascertain (a) why the individual is functioning a certain way, and (b) what the relationship is between such actions and the client's problems. In the first example, what is it about the situation that makes the individual feel guilty? Guilt is subjectively determined with idiosyncratic meaning; therefore, it must be understood from the individual's frame of reference. In the second case, why would the individual rather not go on vacation with his wife and her parents, and why is he unable to handle the situation? Complete understanding—not a solution—is the therapist's task at the beginning of intervention. The therapist should not ask the client in the second case if he has expressed his feelings to his wife or her parents about going on vacation before the therapist understands why it is a problem. Most people in crisis can solve their own problems if emotional interference or inner conflicts are removed from cognitive functioning and the environment facilitates resolution.

To be able to determine the cause of the individual's problem, a therapist must acquire a theoretical understanding of habitual patterns of psychosocial functioning and an understanding of what at present causes the ineffective personality functioning; that is, understanding the meaning of the precipitating event according to the person in crisis. As we have emphasized, achieving this goal necessitates the application of a theoretical perspective.

STEPS FOR WORKING WITH PERSONS IN CRISIS

We now have a frame of reference for our discussion of how to help people resolve crises and become functional again. We will divide this process into steps to make it easier to remember. To become a competent crisis therapist, you must be able to gauge the completeness of your intervention. Knowing the steps of the process helps you make that judgment. Furthermore, working with people in crisis has two parts: an intellectual process and an empathic process. The empathic process is generally the easiest; it is furthered by the client's vulnerability and need for help. The intellectual process is more difficult because it occurs at the same time as the empathic process. This means that the therapist must think at the same time that he or she is feeling and reacting emotionally. Learning by procedural steps helps to develop the intellectual process; the steps provide a cognitive road map for intervention. (Some beginning therapists do not know what to do after the opening greeting because they are not yet familiar with the steps of intervention.) The intervention techniques represent a continuum of interaction in which a therapist uses self, knowledge, and skills to help an individual resolve a crisis and improve social functioning. Bear in mind, however, that these orderly procedures are not rigidly fixed; at times they overlap. The nine procedural steps for helping people in crisis are:

Step 1. Rapidly establish a constructive relationship
Step 2. Elicit and encourage expression of painful feelings and emotions
Step 3. Discuss the precipitating event
Step 4. Assess
Step 5. Formulate a dynamic explanation
Step 6. Restore cognitive functioning
Step 7. Plan and implement treatment
Step 8. Terminate
Step 9. Follow up

Step 1: Rapidly Establish a Constructive Relationship

The process of establishing a relationship is discussed at great length in chapter 4. To review, the therapist should keep in mind the preinterview conditions. The person in crisis is not only suffering and struggling with his or her own problems but may also have feelings about having to turn to a stranger for help. This point was illustrated in the case of Joanne (see chapter 1), who felt that her deceased husband would consider her weak if he knew that she was seeking outside help. The time between the onset of the crisis and the request for help varies greatly. During this time, the individual in crisis is struggling to resolve the crisis without help. Finally having to call someone for help means that the individual cannot resolve the problem alone. The client goes through a process of "giving up" in anticipation of help. Between the request for help and the first appointment, the client will again have to manage alone, even though the request for help can be a source of strength. However, the greater the time between the request for help and the first appointment, the greater the opportunity for distortion and confusion regarding the precipitating event (Kalis et al., 1961).

The major task of the therapist at this point is to appear to the client as a helpful person. This means that the therapist must feel genuine respect for the client as a human being. The client should be greeted with respect, acceptance, and eagerness. Last names with appropriate prefixes should be used, unless the client gives only his or her first name.

It should be remembered that the person in crisis generally feels frightened and often hopeless. He or she has lost the sense of mastery over self and the condition. Self-esteem is generally low. The client may or may not be trying to compensate or save face. The therapist must be sensitive to his or her own initial effect, which may reflect the client's low self-esteem (e.g., using first names before the client is ready). If there is a long walk between the waiting room and the therapist's office, the therapist must be wary of small talk. This is a serious situation, and silence between the waiting room and the therapist's office is more effective than trying to fill the time with artificial small talk. Perhaps the most important aspect of the therapist's task at this point is being sensitive to the client's feelings about seeking help, about the helplessness of the client's condition, and the degree of debilitation. The therapist should be responsive to the client's dependency needs, since they are generally heightened by needing to turn to another for help. In addition, sometimes people in crisis may seek help but feel very pessimistic about the prognosis. Initially they may need reassurance that they can be helped or that they are in the right place. They might say, "I don't know if you can help me," or "I don't know if I'm in the right place or not." In such cases the therapist can respond by saying, "Let's discuss your situation first and then decide what we can do." Still other people in crisis may present the message, "Here I am, take care of me." In such cases the therapist must communicate to the client the feeling that the situation is not hopeless and that by working together something can be done about it. These situations require the therapist to motivate the client. The therapist must use whatever capacities the client has available at the time. To do this, the therapist uses those capabilities of the client that are not affected or are the least affected by the crisis. For instance, sometimes anger can be used as a motivating force. Consider the case of Doug (see chapter 2), who flunked his doctoral comprehensive examinations. His anger could be used as a motivating force if the therapist says something like, "It seems to me that your committee was setting you up to see how motivated you really are. The way you are handling this situation, it will appear to them that you tend to give up very easily. Is this what you want them to conclude?" Such a statement would, of course, be based on a careful assessment, with some notion that what is said will be effective; this might not be a very good motivating statement for the severely depressed, the self-defeating, or the masochistic. The very masochistic person would probably say, "See, you think I'm no good, too." Whatever the therapist says should be purposeful and predicated on knowledge and needs of the client. Still other individuals approach therapy with ambivalent feelings about the helping process for various reasons. Some may feel hopeless—that, since they cannot help themselves, no one else can either. There is also at times a competitive striving in which a client dares someone to help. The client may be ambivalent about the whole process because of rumors or heresay (i.e., what friends, TV, or the press say about therapy). In addition, the client may be worried about what will happen to him at the crisis center or what he will find out about himself. The latter is less of a problem in crisis therapy than in traditional therapy, but nevertheless it occurs, as we saw in the case of Joanne (see chapter 1). To establish a relationship rapidly, the therapist must be sensitive to these possibilities. In traditional therapy the therapist does not have to anticipate as much, since there is time to wait and see what manifests itself. The time required to establish a constructive relationship can be decreased by the therapist's anticipation coupled with the helplessness and need of the client as manifested and revealed in the communication process.

Another factor important in rapidly establishing a constructive relationship is the client's expectations of the helping person. The client no doubt comes to the interview with a preconceived idea or image of the therapist. It may be based on the client's own notions and feelings about helping professionals, on TV images, or on just plain self-esteem. A client may expect to see a younger person, an older person, a shorter person, a taller person, a man or a woman, a psychiatrist, a psychologist, or a medical doctor. The point is that the therapist must be sensitive and perceptive to the client's fears, misgivings, misunderstanding, and lack of knowledge. These can block a constructive relationship and must be dealt with before the client and therapist establish the kind of relationship that is conducive to the goals of crisis treatment. You might not think that a person in crisis would be concerned about some of these factors, but people can be proud to their last breath, even when it is an obstacle to being helped. Consequently such obstacles must be worked through very quickly. This requires a therapist who is not easily threatened or intimidated, one who has confidence in his or her ability and who can accurately interpret human communications.

Understanding is the key to accepting the client as he or she is and not needing to react with judgmental attitudes and behaviors. Consider the following illustration:

Therapist: Hello. I am Mr. Phillips.
Client: Hello. I am Connie Fleming.

Therapist: Will you tell me how you see your problems?
Client: You look pretty young to be a psychiatrist.
Therapist: I'm not a psychiatrist. Were you expecting to see a psychiatrist?
Client: Yes. They told me at the emergency room that psychiatrists were on duty here.
Therapist: I am a psychiatric social worker, and if you're willing to discuss your concerns with me, we can determine whether you need a psychiatrist or whether you and I can work things out.

In this case the therapist is not offended or defensive but is confident in his ability and communicates this confidence to the client. Some clients, regardless of condition, feel that they must have the "best," or the highest-status professional. Nonmedical therapists must deal with this attitude. Sometimes these feelings are based on self-esteem, other times on their feelings about how bad off they are. Still other times it is lack of knowledge about the helping professions. Remember that a long explanation of the differences between various helping professions serves very little, if any, purpose; the client will not generally remember it anyway. What is necessary in such a situation is a simple statement of the professional identity of the therapist, and an exploration of the basis of the client's feelings about working with the therapist. All of this done in a confident and accepting manner helps establish the constructive relationship quickly. The therapist's goal of seeking to understand the client regardless of behavior helps to minimize behavior of the client that could be considered to be a personal attack on the therapist.

Rapidly establishing a constructive relationship is achieved by the therapist's accepting the client, communicating this acceptance through affective and other nonverbal behavior, projecting a genuine interest and natural eagerness to help the client, and feeling confident in the ability to understand and help the client. But how do you know when a constructive relationship has been established? First, the client feels comfortable with the therapist and speaks relatively freely and in a way consistent with what is expected in the crisis condition. For example, a depressed client may not speak completely freely, but within the limits of the condition will respond to a genuine interest and concern. Other signs of a constructive relationship are mutually positive feelings and the client's beginning identification with the therapist, especially with therapeutic goals. In effect, a good relationship is established with the person in crisis when he or she is willing to accept the therapist as an alter ego or self. When signs of a constructive relationship are not apparent, the therapist should find out why.

Step 2: Elicit and Encourage Expression of Painful Feelings and Emotions

Although this step is closely associated with discussing the precipitating event, it is discussed separately here because many beginning therapists miss it in the effort to quickly get to the "facts," the precipitating event. This is a particular problem of the beginning therapist. The precipitating event and significant aspects of the client's life should not be explored until painful feelings and emotions are thoroughly ventilated and are actively flowing. Very often, a client will be visibly upset upon entering the therapist's office—crying, angry or abusive, distraught, or depressed. It is highly therapeutic for the client to ventilate these very strong emotions in a supportive, non-judgmental atmosphere. The therapist should support and encourage their expression before attempting to get to the reason for these feelings. There are other times, however, when clients may seem very controlled as a result of having tried to resolve the crisis themselves. If so, the event itself may be discussed, during which time the painful feelings may surface. When they do, the therapist should encourage their expression. Almost all people in crisis come to the first session manifesting some painful or distressful affect. (If they do not, they are either not in crisis or they are suppressing appropriate crisis affect, or it is a sign of a different problem). The client should be encouraged to express these feelings before moving to the precipitating event. Consider this example:

Therapist: Hello, I'm Ms. Fox.
Client: Hello, I'm Pat Knight.
Therapist: Please tell me what bothers you, Ms. Knight.
Client: *(depressed and crying)* My best friend told me I should come here.
Therapist: I can see that you are very upset. Can you tell me what you are feeling right now?
Client: I'm feeling sad, lonely, and empty—like nobody cares about me.
(NOTE: An expression of feeling "empty" generally means a feeling of being unloved and lonely).

Here the therapist encouraged expression of the painful feelings. After sufficiently expressing the painful feelings, the client can be easily guided to their cause. Following the sequence above:

Therapist: Now tell me, what is causing you to feel the way you do?

Eliciting and encouraging painful feelings lets the individual in crisis gain mastery over overwhelming feelings. The client now faces them with the support of the therapist. A thorough expression of emotions not only facilitates mastery over affect but is also a source of ego restrengthening and the beginning of cognitive restoration. This is achieved through the therapist's skillful encouragement and guidance toward ventilation of feelings and toward thinking in order to respond to the therapist's supportive questions. To encourage a client to express painful feelings, the therapist must use questions that elicit feelings. For example, for the client who feels he or she is falling apart, the therapist needs to know what this feels like. Such statements are based on feelings that need to be explored. Consider the following statement by Menninger (1963):

> The man who feels himself "falling apart" or "going to pieces" has some vague sense of the unity and integrity of his personality. He feels rather than knows this to be a normal or ideal characteristic of life. By "being upset" or unbalanced or "going to pieces," he describes by implication an awareness of an equilibrium which we may well call "the vital balance."

Hence a response would be, "Can you tell me what this feels like?" or "Can you describe for me what this feels like?" This kind of exploration helps the client talk about what it feels like to fall apart, and it can be associated with something more concrete. It also helps the therapist understand what the client means and whether it is real or a figure of speech. Most important, it facilitates empathy, providing the therapist with something to relate to and identify with. Consider this case excerpt:

Therapist: Hi! My name is Jack Stein. Can you tell me what brings you here?
Client: The nurse brought me here. I can't do my job. I feel like I'm falling apart.
Therapist: What do you mean by falling apart?
Client: This happened about a year ago. My girlfriend and I were having problems. I took my ring back because she did not do what I wanted her to, and then I tried to kill myself by cutting my wrist.
Therapist: Is that similar to what's going on now?

In this case, the therapist did not explore what falling apart really feels like for this individual, and the client associated it with a previous experience. Even if the therapist did not explore with the individual what it feels like to be falling apart, we can get some idea by following the client's associations. To this client, "falling apart" means attempting suicide. At this point we cannot be sure that this is what he meant to say, but that is how he responded to the question "What do you mean by falling apart?" This would be a good opportunity to use the technique of clarification; for example, "Are you saying that when you have this feeling like you are falling apart, that is when you attempt to take your own life?" This is also the beginning of some cognitive restoration, because the therapist has asked a causal connecting question. It is also information for assessment and evaluation. Exploring feelings also enables the therapist to better understand what the client is feeling; he or she can empathize with the client's description. The techniques used during this step include ventilation, encouragement, clarification, questioning, exploring, and listening.

There are times when people in crisis may not want to face painful feelings. They may want to handle them by denial or suppression. In such cases, the use of suggestion, reassurance, and universalization may be helpful. For example, a therapist might find it helpful to say, "I know you have said that you want to forget about what has happened to you because it makes you feel worse; but if you can face your feelings about it with me now, it will be better for you in the long run." Or, "Bringing your feelings out in the open is always better than keeping them inside, all alone." Universalization is used much less often than other techniques to initiate and maintain a person's expression of feelings, but sometimes it is useful to let a client know that the expression of the kind of feelings he or she is experiencing is not only necessary but common to all people going through what the client is going through (or has gone through).

The need to encourage a person in crisis to express painful feelings and emotions before moving on to other steps cannot be overemphasized. It requires patience and the capacity to tolerate painful feelings. This is another problem of the beginning therapist. It is very easy to avoid or shorten this step in eagerness to relieve the client of suffering or to move from painful feelings to acts, but the therapist must actually participate in the expression of these feelings through encouraging, eliciting, questioning, exploring, and clarifying such feelings and emotions.

Step 3: Discuss the Precipitating Event

Following a thorough discussion of painful feelings and emotions, the therapist moves to the causes of these feelings—the precipitating event. Recall that crisis theory assumes that social functioning is a continuous activity of maintaining and reestablishing equilibrium in the face of daily upsetting internal and external events. This homeostatic process is achieved through the functioning of the individual's psychic system, and through specific coping mechanisms and habitual patterns of adaptation. Only when some event is perceived to be so threatening to the individual that he or she cannot cope as effectively as before the event does a crisis develop. It follows, therefore, that the therapist should find out what this event is, when it occurred, how it occurred, the circumstances surrounding it, and as much information leading up to the event as needed to understand the individual in crisis. For example, it would be very enlightening in a bereavement crisis to know the nature of the relationship between the client and the deceased, certainly immediately before the death as well as historically. In other situations it is important to know how the client contributed to the occurrence of the precipitating event and what it means. If we recall the case of Ben (see chapter 2), we can see why this is so significant. In Ben's case, the precipitating event was his wife leaving him after he beat her.

It is also very important for the therapist to ascertain how the client has tried to resolve the crisis and how the client has been trying to cope since its occurrence. Most important, the therapist should determine what made the client finally seek help. The therapeutic benefit of discussing the precipitating event, its meaning, and the circumstances surrounding it, is inestimable. It not only provides for emotional release, but it facilitates cognitive restoration and is the basis for assessment and evaluation, as we shall see later. However, ascertaining the precipitating event is not always easy. Sometimes it requires considerable search on the part of the therapist and the client. This is especially true when the individual is very upset or when a series of significant events occur at the same time or in succession. This is illustrated in the case of Alice, who had a series of traumas in a short period of time. She was unmarried and pregnant and had been rejected by her boyfriend. Her mother hated the boyfriend and had obtained a lawyer to force him to pay medical expenses. Further compounding her problem, her mother died unexpectedly.

In cases of multiple problems, the therapist must search for the one event that is the primary cause of the crisis. In Alice's case it became apparent that the boyfriend's rejection and her uncertainty about keeping her baby were the actual precipitating events. Alice did not mention her mother's death until near the end of the interview. However, given a series of successive events, without adequate exploration and clarification of feelings, we would still not be certain which is the precipitating event (the straw that broke the camel's back). The most important event to the client in cases of successive events is generally reflected in present affect and feelings. This is why a thorough exploration of feelings and causes should be completed before the therapist moves to the facts of precipitating events. Regardless of how difficult it is to discover, it is a premise of crisis therapy that a precipitating event invariably exists. It is not unusual for the client to be unable to sort out the precipitating event in this chainlike process. Furthermore, people in crisis generally do not seek help immediately after the precipitating event; consequently, it is not unusual for the individual in crisis to be unable to identify the precipitating event readily. The therapist may need to discuss events and circumstances that took place several weeks before the onset of the crisis.

Discussion of the precipitating event properly starts after painful feelings and emotions have been ventilated. These feelings are an integral part of the therapeutic session. Specific attention should be given to the manner in which the individual in crisis accounts for difficulties. The manner used to describe difficulties can be more revealing than the words used. The key is to stay with the client in his or her emotional state and inquire about the precipitating event simply as a part of it. If the client is inconsistent and illogical, interviewing techniques should be used to help him or her clarify feelings, perceptions, and thinking. As Menninger (1963) states:

> No one can know all of the reasons for his behavior, and yet almost anyone can give many reasons for specific acts. Over and beyond the reasons he gives, there are many reasons which he doesn't give. There are reasonable but unmentioned reasons, and there are unmentioned and unreasonable reasons, reasons depending upon emotions or biological processes of which the individual has no full knowledge.

At this time also, recurring patterns, what is expressed and what is unexpressed, should be observed. Self-defeating or self-punishing behavior characteristics should also be observed. In discussing the precipitating event, the client reveals his or her psychic functioning.

Although it may seem simple, it can be difficult in practice to maintain the emotional flow as the client is moved to discuss the precipitating event. Consider the following interview with Alice.

Therapist: What is your name?
Client: Alice.
Therapist: Hi, Alice, what brings you in today?
Client: *(tearfully)* My lawyer made the appointment. He thought I should come and talk with someone.
Therapist: Your lawyer?
Client: Yes. He made the appointment; he told me to come here.
Therapist: He feels you need to talk to somebody. How do you feel about that?
Client: I guess so *(sigh)*.
Therapist: What is it that you feel that you need to talk about?
Client: *(tearfully, long silence)* I don't know.
Therapist: Confused about what you feel?
Client: *(sobbing)* Yes.

It can be seen that this therapist did not encourage Alice to express painful feelings in spite of the fact that she was obviously upset and in distress. Neither did the therapist search for the precipitating event. The question about the lawyer making the appointment may have been appropriate for a captive client such as a juvenile delinquent sentenced to see a therapist or a school administrator who has told parents that their child cannot come back to school until he or she has gone to the child guidance clinic. In this case, however, we are interested in what the lawyer observed about the client to recommend that she come to the crisis center, since she was not aware of the need herself. The next question should have been, "What do you think are your lawyer's reasons for sending you here?" A more effective approach, however, would have been for the therapist to first recognize the client's upset and encourage her to express these painful feelings, followed by exploring the causes of these feelings. Consider another example that has been discussed before in which a therapist did not explore feelings:

Therapist: Hi! My name is Jack Stein. Can you tell me what brings you here?
Client: The nurse brought me here. I can't do my job. I feel like I'm falling apart.
Therapist: What do you mean by falling apart?

The therapist should have said, "Tell me what that feels like," and should have followed that with ascertaining what was causing the client to feel like he was falling apart, and if he had ever fallen apart before and under what circumstances.

By examining these two interviews, you can see that eliciting and encouraging the expression of painful feelings and determining the precipitating event are not simple tasks.

There are three possible reasons why a therapist has difficulty with these steps: (a) the therapist is avoiding the painful feelings in the client, (b) the therapist is trying to get facts too quickly, or (c) the therapist needs more practice functioning intellectually and empathically at the same time. These two examples also illustrate how the therapist's opening comments set the stage for the remainder of the session. Since crisis is an affective state, opening comments should be formulated to bring out feelings and emotions first, followed by events and information.

Historical Information. Gathering feelings, experiences, and facts about the client's past life is very therapeutic even for the person in crisis. Lewis (1973) most adequately expresses the value of historical information. He states:

> A skillfully taken history can have the effect of holding a mirror up to the patient, thereby helping him to develop a much clearer picture of himself as an historical being than he had before. He may be compelled to look at certain recurrent problems in his life which he has not been able to look at before by reason of denial or cognitive disorganization. A careful history, with persistent questioning as to the patient's feelings about life events, and motivation for life decisions, may lay bare a pattern that he cannot avoid facing for the first time in his life. He may become aware, for example, of patterns of recurrent failure or self-destructiveness, a tendency to regard himself as a passive victim of circumstances, a tendency to create problems for himself, or a tendency to blame others for his inadequacies.

It should be clear that historical information is obtained in the context of the crisis and not as a separate entity. As the individual mentions past events, parents, and so forth during the course of the session, historical information is gathered. The information gathered in this way helps in understanding the basic personality of the individual, the relationship between the past and present, and the assessment and evaluation. The therapist should also observe the attitude associated with the information. Although historical information may appear to be objective, it is always loaded with feelings that are more therapeutic when offered in the context of the crisis. If it is not at least somewhat emotional, the therapist should regard this as significant. For instance, in the case of Alice, the death of her mother was not revealed until some 45 minutes into the session. Until that time she appeared to be distressed only about not knowing what to do about her boyfriend's rejection of her pregnancy. The therapist did not direct her into the causes of her distress. As we move into the assessment and evaluation phase, remember that the therapist must have enough information about the nature of the crisis, the precipitating event, and the life of the client that all significant questions about the client can be answered. This is necessary for assessment and evaluation, especially for identifying the nuclear problem.

Thus, while discussing the precipitating event and searching for the nuclear problem, historical information that lets the therapist understand the individual's usual coping mechanisms and patterns of adaptation can also be ascertained. The following outlines some historical information helpful in understanding, assessing, and evaluating a person in crisis.

Current life situation

A. Interpersonal relationships
  1. Marriage or other long-term heterosexual relationship
    a. How did they meet? What was the attraction?
    b. How long did they know each other before marriage? What was their relationship while dating?

   c. Try to learn some feelings about spouse.
   d. Ascertain any changes in marriage or personality of respective spouse.
   e. Attempt to ascertain feelings about significant others (e.g., love relationships, friends).
  2. Family, children
B. Employment
  1. What, where, how long, degree of functioning, satisfaction.
  2. Relationship with co-workers, supervisor.
C. Background information
  1. Number of siblings and line of birth. Place of birth. Childhood experiences. Developmental facts if unusual, accidents, significant events, separations. Unusual childhood illnesses or the typical ones if there was some adverse effect.
D. Parents (discuss mother and father separately)
  1. Relationship and feelings about parents; childhood memories of them. Take particular notice of how the client describes each parent's personality and how the client feels he or she was treated by each parent.
  2. Nature of parents' relationship. How parents got along with each other. Were they happy? If not, why not? How did the client feel about parents' feelings about their marriage?
  3. Education: how much, how functioned, undue difficulty with any teacher. Activities in school, dating (ascertain parents' feelings about dating). Activities at college.

Not all of this information may be needed, but often much of it is necessary for a complete understanding of the individual and the nuclear problem and to ascertain the client's usual level of social functioning. It is presented here as a guide to some areas that might be explored for better understanding of the individual in crisis. There are, of course, times when the therapist does not have time to gather all of this information, especially in the first interview. However, the more that is known about the client, the better the therapist is able to help. For example, if a person was abandoned or threatened with abandonment in childhood, a current situation may reactivate those old fears. When this happens, the perception and reactions to the previous experiences replace current reality, which generally compounds the problem. It is generally not possible to solve current problems with past unresolved methods and coping mechanisms. Again, historical information is only necessary in relationship to the crisis and as needed to understand the individual's psychosocial functioning. When it is needed, much of this information can be obtained very quickly and therapeutically when the therapist stays affectively where the client is. A discussion of history is most therapeutic when the client is helped to relate the present to the past when it is appropriate.

In sum, thorough exploration and information gathering about the precipitating event should provide the therapist with answers to the following questions:

1. What happened?
2. When did it happen?
3. Where did it happen?
4. How did it happen?
5. What were the circumstances?
6. What were the factors?
7. What was client reaction?
8. How has client been trying to cope or resolve the situation?
9. Has anything like this ever happened to the client before? If yes, how was it handled?
10. How has the client handled other problems in life?
11. If there have been other problems, what is different about this situation?

Answers to these questions should provide the therapist with extensive information about the nature of the precipitating event and the quality of the individual's functional behavior in that situation under specific circumstances. They should also provide information about the person's relationships with significant others.

Step 4: Assess and Evaluate

Assessment and evaluation really begins with the first contact with the client. However, by the time the therapist "officially" reaches this step, he or she has observed the client, listened attentively, elicited and encouraged the expression of painful feelings and emotions, identified and explored the cause and meaning of the precipitating event, and obtained sufficient information about the client, his interpersonal relationships, and other significant aspects of his life. At this point the therapist must systematically use this information to assess and evaluate the client's current level of functioning and capacity for future functioning and to determine some understanding of the client's usual habitual level of functioning. This information becomes the basis for treatment planning and implementation. In sum, during assessment and evaluation the therapist draws conclusions regarding the cause of the individual's crisis, the degree of debilitation, and the potential for recovery.

Determining the Cause of the Crisis Condition. Recall that the cause of the crisis is not specifically the precipitating event but the reaction to the event. Hence the first step in determining the cause of the crisis is for the therapist to identify the nuclear problem. The nuclear problem differs from the precipitating event or present problem. The precipitating event is the way the client perceives and reacts to the current situation. It is of necessity a subjective view of distress and is contaminated by cognitive debilitation, distorted perception, and emotional confusion as a consequence of trying to resolve the crisis alone. It can be compared with trying to repair a television set with hundreds of tubes without knowing how. Although you try to remove all of the tubes at the same time in an orderly fashion, putting them back in the right place is complex. Once you get one out of place, they all become confused and your problems are compounded. Finally the television set blows up, and a professional television repairman has to be consulted.

The nuclear problem, on the other hand, is the underlying reason that causes the individual's reaction to the precipitating event. Burgess and Baldwin (1981, p. 78) also state:

> Many emotional crises are determined, at least in part, by unresolved conflicts or traumas from the past that are reactivated or brought again to awareness by a particular event. The psychodynamic component of the crisis, the precipitant (Hoffman and Remmel, 1975), is frequently instrumental in producing a failure to cope and impedes adaptive crisis resolution unless addressed as part of the crisis intervention process.

It is really the client's unknown personal meaning given to the precipitating event.

In effect, our understanding of anxiety and depression and their derivatives gives us a foundation for understanding the nuclear problem. As we said in chapter 2, almost all reactions to crises are manifested by anxiety, depression, or their derivatives. So the behavioral and affective manifestations of the person in crisis locate the area of the nuclear problem. For example, we know that depression results from (a) loss or threatened loss of a loved object or other ego value; (b) loss or threatened loss of self-concept or self-esteem; (c) the failure to live up to internalized expectations, standards, values, or goals; or (d) the violation or wish to violate some significant moral code (i.e., to engage in or the desire to engage in something personally unacceptable). Although this understanding locates the area, the specific problem is the meaning to the client of the behavioral or affective manifestations. Consider the case of Ben (see chapter 2), who became depressed and suicidal after his wife left him because he beat her. What is the specific meaning of his depression to him? Is it the loss of a loved object that threatens him? Or is it the loss of self-esteem? Since Ben contributed greatly to the precipitating event, it is logical to conclude that he had some wish for his wife to leave. If so, why did he get depressed and react as if he were hurt by the loss of his wife? A possible answer is that he felt considerable conflict over loving his wife versus loving his mother. The conflict could be resolved by his wife leaving him. On the other hand, going to live with his mother was consciously unacceptable. Because he attempted suicide, it is logical to conclude either that this conflict made him feel contemptuous of himself or that the suicidal gesture was symbolically directed at another person, probably his mother or his wife. (As Freud stated, every suicide is a homicide.) Consider the case of Kay, an attractive 35-year-old woman, who developed a crisis when her husband's employer arranged a working retreat at a famous resort for only the executives of the company. Kay felt strongly that the spouses should go also. The precipitating event occurred while she was vociferously expressing her feelings to her husband, who communicated to her both affectively and behaviorally that he did not want her to go. He was in support of his boss; he wanted to go with "the boys." Although Kay complained of the "fear" of being left alone (Kay was not left alone; she had a 14-year-old son at home), the nuclear problem was a deep feeling of rejection and loss of self-esteem because her husband did not want her to go, and on the other hand, she was concerned about her husband's faithfulness. This was supported by Kay's talk about having an affair herself, which was a retaliatory defense against the loss of self-esteem she associated with the possibility of her husband's having an affair, and a fear of herself because the possibility of her having an affair was threatening.

A reliable way to find the nuclear problem is to determine the underlying meaning of the reaction to the precipitating event. Anxiety and depression provide the beginning. The therapist should be careful to look for the sometimes multiple meanings and purposes the nuclear problems serve. As we saw in the case of Ben and Kay, many unacceptable feelings of desire previously handled by keeping them out of conscious awareness can be reactivated by certain external events. When this happens, unacceptable feelings of desire must be defended against or controlled. In Ben's case, he wanted to live with his mother but needed his wife so he could defend against this desire. There are times that the nuclear problem may be tied to the nature of the individual personality and developmental history. In such situations the precipitating event reactivates a previous forgotten conflict. When this happens, the individual reacts to the current crisis in the same way he or she reacted to the old conflict.

These situations respond very well to cognitive restoration. Although we are suggesting areas that can be explored, in order to understand people, the therapist should be interested in gathering meaningful information that is germane to understanding the individual and his or her problems. But we should also keep in mind that discussion of significant historical information, especially that of interpersonal relationships, is very therapeutic.

Assessing Degree of Functional Debilitation. An assessment of the seriousness of the individual's crisis condition and capacity for social functioning can be made as soon as the precipitating event and the nuclear problem are understood.

Before the crisis, the individual was able to use the capacities of the psychic system: intelligence, perception, judgment, and so forth. The client related and adapted to the social environment. The crisis interrupted these processes. We are interested at this point in which of the functions have been interrupted and to what degree. We are interested also in those functions that are not impaired or that are the most functional.

The first step in assessing the seriousness of the individual's crisis state is to observe and estimate the degree of debilitating affect or emotions: depression, anxiety, and their derivatives. The therapist should get answers to such questions as: How depressed does the individual seem? How anxious? How angry? Is he or she homicidal or suicidal? Remember that the greater the depression, the greater the internalized anger. As a general rule, the deeper the depression, the less likelihood there is of suicide; the depression immobilizes the individual because of the anger that is turned inward. Consequently, the danger of suicide for the depressed is not during the depth of the depression, but while going into and coming out of the depression, when the individual has more energy. Thus far, we have been discussing the assessment of basically normal crisis reactions. Expanding the crisis model to include serious mental health conditions means that the crisis therapist must be prepared to work in all settings and to treat violent and psychotic behavior in addition to treating normal crisis conditions. Suicide and homicide will be discussed further in chapter 6. It should suffice for the time being to say that when either of those subjects are brought up by the client, either subtly or directly, the therapist must rule out, through exploration, the potentiality of its occurrence. The therapist should be satisfied that the suicide or homicide is not likely to occur before the client leaves the office; otherwise, the therapist should offer the client protective measures such as hospitalization.

All mental disorders are divided into two classes: organic and functional; in the discussion of assessment it is important to differentiate between them (Levy, 1982). Organic mental disorders are those with a known cause related either to structural damage or operational malfunction of the brain (Levy, 1982). The kind of disease process that falls under this heading is a condition such as that seen in some elderly patients whose mental disturbances are related to structural changes in the brain. Organic mental disorders also include all disorders that have as their cause a demonstratable metabolic disturbance in the body (Levy, 1982). Examples are the emotional and behavioral changes associated with chronic renal disease and hypothyroidism. Disorders of emotion, thought, and behavior caused by intoxication or withdrawal from a drug, or that result from the effect of continued excessive use of a substance, are also considered organic mental disorders. The functional disorders category contains all of the mental disorders for which there is not yet a well-established structural or metabolic cause (Levy, 1982).

The distinction between functional and organic disorders is a very important one for the crisis therapist. It lets the therapist know immediately if a referral to a medical specialist is necessary. Such a knowledge enables the therapist to discuss with any involved family members the treatment and prognosis of the problem. The procedure for assessing psychosis and degree of debilitation is the Mental Status Examination with which every crisis therapist should be familiar.

The overwhelming effect of emotions on the functions of the psychic system determines the degree of functional debilitation. Hence to find the client's capacity for social functioning resulting from overwhelming emotionality, the degree of debilitation of the various functions of the psychic system must be assessed.

The functions of the psychic system that make possible unique and idiosyncratic social functioning and adaptation are cognitive functioning, perception, memory, reality testing, judgment, thought processes, impulse control, adaptive efforts, and coping mechanisms. By assessing these various functions and capacities of the psychic system, the therapist not only identifies the impaired functions, but they become a focus of treatment, reinforcement, and restrengthening. Again, the functions of the psychic system are an integrated whole, and some overlap. They are separated here for the sake of study and learning.

Cognitive Functioning. By cognitive functioning we do not mean IQ. We mean the use of information processing, thinking ability, perception, memory, planning, and problem-solving methods. An estimate of the level of cognitive functioning can be determined through several clues: (a) the methods the individual uses to try to resolve the crisis; (b) the adequacy and consistency in discussing events preceding the onset of the crisis; (c) the logic and consistency with which facts and reasons are discussed; and (d) the capacity to comprehend, understand, and make logical responses to the therapist's questions and explanations. We know from the nature of a crisis that these cognitive functions will be impaired to varying degrees. Hence we are interested in evaluating the degree. We are also interested in assessing the individual's capability to receive, digest, and interpret new information. This provides some estimate of how much cognitive capacity has been restored.

Reality Testing. Reality testing is important to adequate social functioning because it requires reconciling the internal world with the events and conditions of the real world. When reality testing is impaired, there is confusion, and in extreme cases, psychosis. Reality testing is the ability to distinguish between what is in the mind and what is in the objective world. In effect, two realities exist in every human being: psychic or subjective reality, that which is in our minds; and objective reality, that which is in the real world. Theoretically, these two realities should be the same; however, this is not always possible. Each person's view of reality is influenced by inner processes, thoughts, imagination, wishes, beliefs, fears, hopes, memories, desires, and experiences. Consequently, it is not easy to consistently see reality objectively. However, adequate social functioning requires a certain degree of success in reality testing. The individual's inner processes must be relatively consistent with objective reality, and he or she must be able to appraise objective reality with some accuracy as the basis for behavior and adaptation. When people are able to test reality successfully, their social functioning is generally good. On the other hand, when reality testing is impaired, what is in the individual's mind is projected onto external reality. Reacting accordingly, that becomes the person's total reality. An example is the individual who develops hallucinations or delusions. He or she reacts as if the delusions are reality. Since the delusions actually contradict reality, the individual develops great problems in social functioning. Psychosis is the extreme form of impaired reality testing. In more common situations, you can probably recall a time where your imagination, projected onto reality, created a seeming nightmare for you. Even more common are the use of magic and superstition as reality, even when objective reality contradicts them.

For the crisis therapist, the concept of reality testing is not only important for assessing, but also for understanding the individual. Consider the example of an individual who says (and does not mean it as a figure of speech), "I'm scared to death of taking beginning tennis lessons." This person has also made the same statement about flying and sickness. Is that person's reality testing impaired? To a certain extent it is, since the same danger is being associated with beginning tennis lessons as with flying and sickness. In other words, the individual projects inner fears onto tennis, which become reality as far as tennis is concerned. Often, the person in crisis does the same thing. Impaired reality testing can be estimated by the degree of inaccuracy or misinterpretation of objective reality.

Whatever is in the person's mind is his or her reality. Although we may want to change it, we first should accept it and feel empathic. Pain and suffering in the mind hurt just as much as they do when they have an objective cause. The husband who feels that his wife does not love him despite objective evidence to the contrary feels just as unloved as if it were true. The physician who is depressed because he feels he did not do all he could to save his patient in the face of evidence to the contrary feels just as bad as if he had neglected something. Very often, making the individual in crisis aware that he or she is reacting to the events of the real world based on psychic reality can be quite effective, *if* the pain has been accepted and empathized with first. Thus, reality testing is used not only as a means to assess capacity for social functioning and understanding the individual in crisis, but also for treatment in cognitive restoration.

The extreme form of impaired reality testing is loss of a sense of reality. This is reflected in psychosis, depersonalization, and the heavy use of drugs.

Perception. Perception is the basis of reality testing and a part of the cognitive process. In simple terms, it is the way an individual sees reality. Of interest, it is based on experience and memory and greatly influenced by specific intraphysic functioning, need, and motivation. It follows, therefore, that perception affects reality testing and judgment.

Impulse Control. Impulse control refers to the ability to control intense emotions and urges (e.g., sexual and aggressive drives). Assessment is especially important to the individual whose anger or aggression could manifest itself in homicide, assaultive behavior, or physical abuse. An example is the individual who is angry at a spouse or child and fears becoming abusive. Perhaps the first factor in assessing an individual whose uncontrolled impulses have been precipitated by a specific event is to estimate the strength of the impulse in relation to the strength of the ego and other countercontrol mechanisms. For example, a person with a relatively strong conscience, though very angry, may be less likely to lose control than a person with a weaker conscience.

A second factor in assessing impulse control is history. People who have a history of poor impulse control are more likely to lose control than people with a history of good control. The exception is the overly controlled or rigid individual. The individual who has a history of rarely getting angry or not showing normal emotions should be evaluated thoroughly, and caution should be taken.

Another factor to be considered in assessing impulse control is the meaning to the individual of the event precipitating the threat of loss of impulse control. Is it loss of self-esteem? Is it personal hurt? Is it perceived as exploitation? Is it taking away something that is an important ego value, for which the individual must take revenge? In those situations, unless the individual has effective counterforces against the impulse, retaliation or loss of control should be a serious consideration.

Another factor is to try to ascertain whether the precipitating event really activated feelings that were meant for another source. For example, a parent battering a child could be having feelings about a sibling or some relationship with his or her own parents.

Not all problems of impulse control involve rage, aggression, or hostility. Sometimes they involve sexual impulses and the threat of unacceptable sexual indulgence or acting out, heterosexually or homosexually. In such situations the therapist must listen carefully to the client. In those situations, if an individual comes for help, it is almost always because there is conflict over the impulse; that is, the desire to indulge versus the feeling that it is wrong. Regardless of how liberal or traditional the therapist is, he or she should not impose personal feelings or views on the client but identify the conflict, hear what the client is asking for, and help the client resolve the conflict. The potentiality and consequence of losing control of impulses other than agressive ones should be thoroughly evaluated also. Specifically, focus should be given to what is provoking the threat of loss of impulse control in all cases.

Thought Processes. Thought processes are important in the assessment when they reveal an incipient psychosis or impending break with reality. In such cases the individual's thought processes may appear to be reasonable but on close scrutiny are either illogical or inappropriate. There may be disproportionate emphasis on something insignificant. Thought may be preoccupied with small physical complaints. Often a client may give specific and exacting details of normally embarrassing subjects, such as sex practices, before he or she really knows the therapist. New words may be used. The client may be distractable and have a poor attention span. Perseveration may be present; that is, the client may persistently repeat an idea or thought. The client may give trivia or irrelevant details about other subjects along with the main point or idea. As though processes progressively deteriorate, they become incoherent and disorganized. The final stage of deterioration is psychosis manifested by delusions, hallucinations, or both, the recognition of which is easy. But recognizing the early stages of psychosis requires a constant sensitivity to the communication process. The therapist must be sure of what the client is saying, and if questions to clarify it do not succeed, serious disturbance in thought processes should be suspected and serious deterioration should be ruled out. Disturbances in thought processes are probably the best indicators of incipient psychosis. As long as an individual's thought processes are understandable or can be made understandable by logical responses to questions, the ego or self-system is reasonably intact.

Effort at Adaptation and Coping Mechanisms. We have seen that through the socialization process people develop habitual patterns of adaptation and coping mechanisms. Under normal conditions these enable them to function and to restore equilibrium when it is upset. In the development of a crisis, both of these break down, forcing the desperate individual to resort to less effective adaptive efforts and coping mechanisms. They are less effective because usual cognitive functions are impaired by overwhelming affect and because the most successful adaptative efforts, the ones habitually used, have become ineffective. It is like a solid foundation moved from under a person, leaving him or her suspended by uncertainty. Given the degree of cognitive impairment, an important index of the degree of debilitation is how the individual is attempting to deal with the crisis. This is a question the therapist must be able to answer. The therapist must also answer the question of what defense or coping mechanisms the client is using. Is the client using the defense mechanisms of projection, denial, reaction formation, or rationalization more than is beneficial? These are mechanisms that keep people from assuming responsibility for their behavior and from facing the reality of the situation. How are they functionally being used? What purpose do they serve? What are the consequences of the client's efforts to deal with the crisis? When greatly regressed, a person relies on primitive beavior patterns. If the therapist can identify the characteristics of these behavior patterns, the level of psychic functioning can be identified. For example, the person who resorts to excessive dependency needs or submissiveness is functioning in a way characteristic of an early phase of life. The impulsive acting-out client is another who is functioning at a level characteristic of early life. It simply means that the ego has become ineffective and that the individual is dominated by emotions. When this occurs it is generally an indication that the therapist must attempt to restore self-control or take active steps to ensure self-control.

In some cases as individual will attempt to deal with the crisis by being overcontrolled. The use of the mechanisms of intellectualization and isolation are examples. Being overcontrolled, in the long run, can often be just as ineffective in consequence to the client as losing control. Consequently, being overcontrolled should not be viewed as being strong, and efforts should be made to help the person deal with the crisis in a therapeutic way; that is, to face it and to express the painful emotions.

Potential for Recovery. The final area to be assessed is the individual's residual capacity to function and to adapt. This evaluation comes at the end of the session with the therapist. By now a great deal of treatment has gone on since the beginning of the session. The client should be different at the end of the session than at the beginning. So the question now is: How integrated is the client? What is his or her capacity to tolerate the effect of the crisis now? How much has ego or cognitive functioning improved? Which of these and other ego functions are operable now? Which are still impaired? To what extent has the client been able to integrate the content of the session? Can the client be sent back to his or her environment until the next appointment?

These questions cannot be answered until the client's external resources have been assessed. These include relatives, significant others, friends, and other helping professionals. Relatives or significant others and external sources of support should be assessed carefully, including the client's feelings about and relationships with them. Some of this may have taken placed while gathering historical information during the affectual release early in the session. Many people are in crisis because of conflict, disappointment, or rejection by significant people in their lives. If the evidence suggests the involvement of others, it should be discussed thoroughly with the client. If the therapist indicates that relatives should be involved and the client is opposed to this suggestion, it should be treated as a form of resistance and worked through if possible. Whether the therapist acts against the client's will depends on the degree of need for involvement of others in the client's crisis, and the consequences if they are not involved. Another factor to consider is the client's right of self-determination, within his or her capacity for reality testing.

The result of the assessment process should enable the therapist to recommend the kind of treatment that will further alleviate the crisis and restore the client's social functioning to at least the precrisis level. To do this, the therapist must be able to synthesize a wealth of information into some understandable causal explanation and then communicate it back to the client in such a way that the client receives, understands, digests, and integrates it.

Step 5: Formulate a Dynamic Explanation

We have conceptualized social functioning as being determined by the psychic system, the array of functions and forces that receives its stimulus for action from both internal and external sources. The word "dynamic" is used to mean the interplay of the functions and forces of the psychic system and the social environment, causing specific ways of social functioning and patterns of adaptation. Hence the therapist must understand and explain the significant forces that are causing the person's crisis condition. The therapist must understand both internal and external factors that precipitated the crisis, as well as those sustaining it and preventing the client from resolving it alone. The dynamic formulation explains certain affective states and identifies specific defense or coping mechanisms, how they are being used, and for what purpose. Through the dynamic formulation, the therapist comes to understand the relationship between the precipitating event and the psychic forces it mobilizes.

The dynamic formulation is the basis of cognitive restoration and treatment planning. It is the basis of client insight and understanding of the crisis condition and reaction. Understanding leads to control and change. There can be no change without understanding. It is also the basis for the type of treatment needed (e.g., crisis therapy or environmental manipulation). In sum, the dynamic formulation is the therapist's understanding of the cause of an individual's reaction to an event precipitating a crisis condition. It is not *what* (e.g., the loss of a loved one) but *why* the client reacts the way he or she does. It establishes the therapist's rationale for how the crisis can be resolved and the client restored to at least a precrisis level of social functioning. It seeks to answer the following questions: What is the core or nuclear problem (i.e., the condition that causes the reaction to the precipitating event)? What is its basic meaning to the client? Why does the client perceive the precipitating event as he or she does? What are the implications to the client's basic personality structure of the meaning of the event and the way he or she tried to resolve the crisis?

Sometimes the dynamic formulation can be made with a minimum of facts and information about the client. At other times it requires a great deal of historical information. Whatever it requires, the therapist must arrive at as accurate a dynamic formulation as possible as the basis of treatment planning and implementation.

Step 6: Restore Cognitive Functioning

A great deal of therapeutic work has gone on before the process of cognitive restoration begins. Generally by this time a person in crisis has gained some relief from painful emotions and tension by expressing them. He or she has begun to use some cognitive facilities again by talking about traumatic experiences and painful feelings. Cognitive faculties have been forced into further use by responses to the therapist's "think" questions. The therapist's effort to thoroughly understand the individual, the nature of the crisis, the nuclear problem, and the significance of the precipitating event have all served this end. Now the client is ready to know what is wrong, why it happened, and what can be done about it. Hence cognitive restoration is the process in which the therapist conveys to the person in crisis an explanation of the causes of the crisis, of the meaning of the nuclear problem, and why the way the individual attempted to handle the crisis was ineffective. Cognitive restoration is an empathic, intellectual process somewhat like a physician's explaining to a patient what is physically wrong. Consider the following example from Walker (1953):

> If on completion of the history and physical examination, the patient is believed to be suffering primarily from an anxiety reaction or psychogenic cardiovascular reaction, he is informed somewhat as follows: "Mr. Jones, after a thorough examination I do not believe you have any serious heart disease, although you have suffered from distressing chest pain and are naturally concerned about it. The pounding and skipping of your heart, I believe, result from a nervous reaction rather than from disease in your heart. For instance, if you walked down a dark alley at night and a masked bandit suddenly stuck a gun in your ribs, I am sure your heart would beat very fast and hard—not because it was bad, but in response to the nerve impulse that went out because of the fear you were experiencing. Your breath would also come short and fast and your hands would be wet and shaking as they were when you come into the office. Prolonged worry, tension, anger, or anxiety can produce the same nervous impulse as intense fear. That this is probably a factor in your case is suggested by the appearance of your symptoms shortly after the arrival of the new foreman with whom you are having trouble. . . . You are afraid that your heart is bad, and as a double check I suggest we get an electrocardiogram, chest x-ray, blood test, and urinalysis as a part of a complete medical evaluation. I expect they will be normal, and, even if they aren't, I am sure most of your symptoms result from nervous causes since no form of heart trouble can completely explain your symptoms, while a tension state readily can."

As McGuire (1965) states:

> Of those patients who eventually gain insight, nearly all begin their own mental ordering and analyses of conflicts in the period between the evaluation and the start of therapy:

Cognitive restoration is needed because the emotional state resulting from the precipitating event is so painful that the client's goal is to avoid or defend against the painful affect, not resolve the crisis. The premise of cognitive restoration is the belief that after a thorough ventilation of feelings, knowledge and understanding will reduce emotional overloading, restore cognitive functioning, and facilitate regaining cognitive control. In other words, by providing an explanation to the client of the reason for the crisis state and the meaning of the behavior, the therapist helps the client to regain mastery of life.

When the therapist has sufficiently completed the first five steps, cognitive restoration is indicated. It generally occurs near the end of the first session, after the therapist has a thorough understanding of the client and the condition and has mentally formulated what is causing the client's problems and why. Cognitive restoration involves the techniques of interpretation and causal connecting explanations. For example, an explanation of the cause of pessimism is presented to the client in simple, clear, and concise statements using words that the client can understand rather than professional jargon. The explanation can be either short or long, depending on the complexity of the client's crisis condition and personality structure. Consider the following cognitive restoration statement:

Fred, a 55-year-old man who three years ago had a laryngectomy, came to the center in a crisis precipitated by his wife's final threat to leave him. For the past four months Fred had felt uncontrollably forced to spend the last three nights of each week "with the boys," nightclubbing, drinking, and having a good time. The other four nights he worked two jobs, rarely coming home before 11 p.m. During the session Fred insisted that he loved his wife and did not want to lose her, as evidenced by his seeking immediate help. When the therapist reached the cognitive restoration phase, he tersely said, "The cause of your condition is that you seem to be living your life as if it is coming to an end soon." Fred eagerly returned for his next session, feeling very pleased with himself. He had returned home to his wife, did not go out with his friends for the weekend, and quit one of his two jobs. Although he returned for two more sessions, he made such a quick recovery that the therapist asked permission to see his wife, who confirmed his change. She was pleased and thought the therapist was a "miracle worker." In follow-up contact with Fred, he was asked what he thought the therapist did that helped him most. He said it was explaining to him that he was living like his life was coming to an end.

It is very difficult to explain all of the variables that made the cognitive restoration phase so significant for Fred. It could have been that perhaps he had some latent feelings of impending death, as he had had cancer. But at the same time his doctor felt that Fred was in good health. The important point is that the therapist's cognitive restoration statement enabled Fred to regain control over his emotions and behavior.

In sum, cognitive restoration helps the client regain control over cognitive faculties and social functioning by providing an explanation of the causes of the crisis condition and an understanding of how and why the client reacted in a particular way.

Step 7: Plan and Implement Treatment

Many crises situations can be resolved in one session. In these cases, no further treatment is necessary and the therapist can move on to termination and follow-up in the first session. In most cases, however, further treatment planning and implementation are necessary.

After the therapist has provided the client with some understanding of the causes and reasons for the crisis condition through cognitive restoration, treatment planning can be recommended. Based on the assessment and evaluation of the client's condition, specific psychic system, and capacity for social functioning, treatment planning is the therapist's professional judgment of what is needed to help the client resolve the crisis and improve social functioning. Specific treatment plans that use the client's motivation, strengths, and capacity should be shared and discussed. The therapist has three basic choices of treatment plans: additional crisis therapy, environmental modification, and referral.

Additional Crisis Therapy. Additional crisis therapy is indicated when the assessment reveals that the individual can safely be treated outside of a hospital but needs additional sessions to further resolve the crisis and restore social functioning.

If additional sessions are indicated, they should be recommended in ways that the client can understand and accept. Using the word "psychotherapy" or other professional jargon should be avoided. Also, a definite appointment should be given at the conclusion of the first session. In other words, the client should not be asked when he or she would like to come back. It should be stated as, "I would like to see you again tomorrow at 10:00 a.m." A recommendation of crisis therapy could be handled like this: "I believe that you and I, through discussions like we had today, can work things out for you. What do you think about that?" Or the therapist might say, "You seem to be feeling better and looking at things differently now, and I would like to have a few more sessions with you like we had today. I would like to see you tomorrow (or next week) at 10:00 a.m. Is that all right?" Or "I think if we can meet a few more times and pursue further some of the things we talked about today, maybe we can make things like they used to be. I can see you on Wednesday at 9:00 a.m. Is that a good time for you?"

If involving significant others is indicated, that recommendation should be stated with confidence, along with an explanation and consideration of the individual's feelings about it. This can be sensitive, since many crises are precipitated by problems with significant others. Assessment of the nature of the client's relationship with significant others and consequences of involving them should be done before the recommendation is made or permission is sought from the client.

Thus far we have been discussing those things that usually happen in the first session. Now more definitive action on the part of both the therapist and the client are set forth in goals established during the treatment-planning process. Keeping within the framework of crisis theory, the individual's crisis should be resolved within the next five weeks. The causes of the crisis state have been identified and thoroughly discussed, and the goals have been laid out and explained to the client in the first session. The therapist can move toward definite action designed to further resolve the crisis, based on an idea of what is causing the crisis. In other words, the cause of the crisis and capacity for social functioning suggest the solution. This indicates that both the therapist and the client become active in the further resolution of the crisis by taking decisive steps to improve psychic functioning. For example, if the client's crisis was the result of a rejection or loss of a love relationship, the client should be encouraged to join clubs or otherwise expand his or her social network. What is discussed in the sessions with the therapist must be applied in reality. The therapist should try to increase the client's self-esteem by supporting the client's ego when it is appropriate and by empathically communcating a feeling that the client has worth. This means that the therapist continues to be sensitive to the client's needs, desires, fears, and conflicts as the client communicates them overtly and covertly. The therapist motivates and encourages, keeping in mind the dictates of psychological support and cognitive restoration. The therapist reinforces strengths and bolsters weaknesses and provides the insight that helps the client regain cognitive control. The therapist does not wait for the client to develop insight, as in traditional psychotherapy; the therapist imparts it personally. Insight occurs through the cognitive restoration process; specifically, through the use of causal connecting statements and interpretation. The success of interpretation is based on three factors: timing, clarity of expression, and the receptiveness of the client. Timing refers to making the interpretation at the most effective point; that is, when it is current in the client's mind and can be connected to current feeling or behavior. It is ineffective to tell that client that he is expecting his wife to treat him the same way as his mother if he is not emotionally feeling it at the time of the interpretation. There must be evidence that he is expecting the same treatment. In other words, there must be some evidence, behaviorally or affectively, to support the basis for the interpretation. The therapist should also elicit the client's interpretation of the meaning of the feelings and behavior, most often before the therapist gives his own.

Clarity of expression refers to the therapist making the interpretation as plainly and succinctly as possible; the shorter and simpler the therapist's statements, the greater their impact. Simetimes the use of parables or analogies is quite effective.

Receptiveness refers to the client's readiness to accept the interpretation. This is usually less of a problem with people in crisis than for those in traditional therapy. People in crisis are generally less defensive. Even so, the therapist should try to anticipate and gauge the effect of the interpretation. The therapist should make sure that the interpretation does not unduly decrease self-esteem. Nor should it be too anxiety-provoking, although an optimal amount of anxiety can be a positive motivating force.

Environmental Modification. Environmental modification involves recommending that the client in crisis be removed from his or her environment because it is impeding improvement or because the client cannot function in it safely. As we saw in chapter 4, there are three basic reasons for recommending environmental modification: (a) the client is incapable of improving as long as he or she remains in the current environment, (b) the client is not able to change the environment constructively, and (c) environmental modification is needed as an adjunct to supportive intervention. Involving significant others is a form of environmental modification.

If hospitalization is indicated, rarely if ever should the client be trusted to report to the hospital alone. Recommending the removal of a child from home or from a foster home is another delicate proposition that should be done only after thorough assessment and evaluation of the situation. This process requires a great deal of knowledge and skill because of the extreme defensiveness of those causing the situation, coupled with society's implication of blame. It is imperative that the therapist in such situations remain as nonjudgmental as possible and recognize even before contact with the client that the therapist will be perceived as a representative of society who is angry, condemning, and punitive ("just wanting to take my child away"). In such situations, the therapist must work through the client's feelings of anticipated blame, defensiveness, resistance, and other negative reactions before real therapeutic work can begin. Regardless of the nature of the crisis, the therapist's purpose is to be helpful.

Step 8: Terminate

After the crisis has been resolved and the individual has returned to the precrisis level of functioning, termination of therapy is indicated. Although crisis therapy is over, the client should have learned from the experience. The client should have learned through the process of self-understanding how to cope better and how to go about solving the next upsetting event, thus preventing a crisis condition. The client should have learned that he or she has ability and capacity, can do something about his or her life, and can live a good life within personal limitations and those of the environment. The client should have learned that he or she must take responsibility for what is wanted, for wanting what is achievable, and for engaging in behavior that will achieve those ends.

Termination should be concluded with the client feeling that the therapist will be there if needed again, as in the case of Joanne (see chapter 1). Knowing that the therapist is available is often a source of support. However, in most bona fide crises, it is rarely needed.

Step 9: Follow-up

At the end of the last session the client should be informed that the therapist will be interested in how the client is getting along and will be in contact at some time in the future. Generally, clients feel good about such interest and welcome the information. Some crisis therapists, however, believe that such a follow-up prolongs dependency feelings, although this has not been proved. The advantages the client gains from this interest usually outweigh questionable negative consequences. Furthermore, such follow-up lends itself to evaluation of results, which becomes the basis of new knowledge for working with people in crisis.

SUMMARY OF THE TREATMENT PROCESS FOLLOWING THE INITIAL SESSION

Sessions following the initial one should start with an exploration of how the client has been feeling and functioning since the last session. Clarification and encouragement should be used to ensure that the client reports as much as possible about the crisis and his or her efforts to effect resolution. The therapist questions and clarifies the client's ways of perceiving, feeling, thinking, and behaving and supports the client when the client needs and is ready to receive such support for the development of positive behavior and efforts. Through the technique of interpretation the therapist helps the client develop insights into unconscious behaviors and obstacles preventing further crisis resolution. After an interpretation, alternative options should be discussed so the client will have something to replace painful feeling and ineffective perceiving, thinking, relating, and behaving.

Interpretations help clients become aware of why they feel and behave the way they do, the meaning of their feelings and behavior, what they hope to gain from their behavior, and why it is ineffective. This self-understanding enables the clients to choose effective means of meeting needs now that they know what these needs truly are. This process is repeated during each of the subsequent sessions until the crisis is resolved, adequate coping is restored, and termination is indicated.

TREATMENT OF PEOPLE IN CRISIS BY GROUP THERAPY

Recently, group therapy has become an accepted method of treatment for people in crisis; however, given the personal and subjective nature of a serious crisis, the individual should be evaluated carefully before being placed in a group. Rarely, if ever, should a person in crisis be placed in a group before the first interview, and only after the client's emotionalism and debilitation are sufficiently reduced. Emotionalism has been sufficiently reduced after the client has shared painful feelings associated with the precipitating event and, in the opinion of the therapist, has begun to think more clearly. The group process is especially beneficial for those in crisis because it offers a social network of support, acceptance, and empathy. The common bond of the crisis enables each member to be supportive of every other member. New perspectives are gained as members share and help others discuss their crisis situations. Interactions and transactions reveal to each client his own ineffective functioning resulting from the crisis. It is often easier to see someone else's problems and offer solutions; group members can develop personal insight as well as gain insight from the feedback of others. Direct action for solving problems is encouraged.

The therapist who initially assesses the client should be the group leader, if possible. By so doing, the therapist can maintain the continuity of an already established and very often intense relationship. Then too, the client does not have to enter the group as a total stranger.

Membership in a group is not new, as most people were born into a group—the family. A group is three or more people who join together for a specific purpose or to accomplish a specific goal. It is characterized by interaction, structure, and the presence of a leader. At least three group members are necessary to ensure interactions. Interactions are determined by the group's purpose, leadership, composition, and structure. There are many types of therapy and psychotherapy groups. Therapy differs from psychotherapy in that the former is goal-directed, here-and-now-oriented, short-term, supportive, and focuses on interpersonal insight development; the latter is usually long-term and emphasizes intrapsychic insight development (Levine, 1979).

Purpose of Crisis Group

A crisis group is intended to achieve basically the same goals as in the therapist/client relationship; namely, (a) to relieve debilitating emotionality such as tension, anxiety, and moderate depression; (b) to help resolve some conflicts that interfere with functioning and contribute to the crisis, (c) to help develop some understanding of the cause and reason for being in crisis, and (d) to return the person to at least the precrisis level of psychosocial functioning. There are several advantages a crisis group offers to both the therapist and the client. First, more people can be seen by the therapist; second, a number of people attempting to solve each problem has the effect of multiple influence. In the case of open group membership, members at later levels of crisis resolution can offer encouragement and hope to new members.

Size and Composition

Careful selection of crisis group members is important. At a minimum, the therapist should complete the assessment in order to reduce emotionality, to establish a relationship, and to prepare the person for group membership. The therapist should explain the purpose, goals and process of the group. The client must be convinced that the group is going to help, so the therapist must allay any fears or resistance. The assessment interview will also help the therapist come to better know the client and to identify information that the client may not want to initially share with "strangers." As previously stated, this interview will also enable the client to feel that at least one person in the group is familiar—the therapist.

The group should be composed of no fewer than four members and no more than eight; six is optimal.

Selection Process

If the therapist sees the person in crisis for one or more assessment interviews in which the effects of the crisis are reduced, selection for group membership can be made at the therapist's discretion. People experiencing crises who are sociable and communicative, and whose goals can be met by the group process, can be placed in a group. However, clients whose crises are precipitated by alcohol or drugs, or those suffering from severe depression or acute psychosis, should not be placed in a group (Satterfield, 1977). As Yalom (1975, 1985) states:

> These patients seem destined to fail because of their inability to participate in the primary task of the group; they soon construct an interpersonal role which proves to be detrimental to themselves as well as to the group. Consider the sociopathic patient, an exceptionally poor risk for outpatient, interactional group therapy. Characteristically, these patients are destructive to the group. Although early in therapy they may become important and active members, they will eventually manifest their basic inability to relate, often with considerable dramatic and destructive impact.

Although Comstock and McDermott (1975) found some success treating suicidal people in group, it is our view that suicidal people should not be put in a group. The pain and disappointment produced by failed love relationships are too great for them to tolerate the scattered relationships and the possibility that the group members may respond to their suicide attempts with anxiety and anger and thus reject them. Furthermore, the suicidal person needs the satisfaction of expressing emotional needs in the security of the individual relationship to help him or her develop and to recognize that life is worth living. Motto (1979), for example, related a negative experience he had as a result of placing a suicidal client in a group:

> In retrospect we felt that her obvious strengths had diminished the sense of urgency (which) her statement should have generated, that her vivacity led us to underestimate the degree of depletion of her emotional energy, and that we were clearly too slow in shoring up her overall support system. One group member had started this task by setting up an outside contact to help her separate her work situation but she did not follow through and it became evident that our effort was too little too late.

Structure of Crisis Groups

Structure refers to group organization and number of times the group will meet as well as how often, how long, and where. Most crisis therapy groups should be open-ended, which means that the group exists on a continuous basis; as one person leaves another fills the vacant space. In contrast, a close-ended group is one that ends when all members terminate; no new members are added.

Time and Place

The crisis group can meet as often as necessary to resolve crises and return the individuals to precrisis levels of functioning. Most crisis groups will meet once or twice per week, although we have found success with 3 three-hour group sessions; this was not consciously predetermined—it just happened to serve the needs of the clients of this particular group. Since the temporal nature of crisis still is the guideline, the group need not last longer than six to eight weeks. Satterfield (1977) and Strubler and Allgeyer (1967) believe that most crisis groups can complete their tasks within four meetings.

Settings

The place of meeting may be determined by the availability of space. However, the setting should be comfortable and large enough to allow everyone to see and interact with everyone else.

Role of Therapist

The role of the therapist in a crisis group is to facilitate group interaction and to maintain group focus on the problem. The therapist must encourage the group to do the "therapy." The therapist guides, directs, facilitates, and interprets. In one group, for example, Mr. Hanover wanted to talk about how difficult his life was with his wife rather than how hurt he was when she left him. The therapist could say, "I wonder why we allow Mr. Hanover to talk about how terrible his wife was rather than how painful her leaving was." This not only emphasizes the need to discuss painful feelings, but reminds the group members of their responsibility to keep problems in focus. The therapist encourages group members to help each other and share their feelings and thoughts.

Problem resolution should be the main focus, and members should be encouraged to share their ideas or solutions; it is often easier to see someone else's problems and possible solutions than it is to see and solve one's own. In response, the therapist must help the group members to recognize and understand the cause and effect of their suggestions.

The Group Process

Rapidly Establish a Constructive Relationship. The therapist should formulate the establishment of a constructive relationship early and encourage group interaction. The first session can begin with a statement to this effect: "We are here because we all have serious problems and we can help each other because it is easier to see someone else's problems than our own."

Focus on the Precipitating Event. After the introduction, the therapist should have each group member discuss the nature and circumstances of their respective precipitating events. If the group members do not ask sufficient questions, the therapist should elicit the expression of painful feelings and emotions, both manifest and submerged.

Assess. The therapist should encourage the group members to share their beliefs regarding the condition of the client and offer support for their views. Very often, when one person states how "bad off" or "how well off" another person is, it can be a challenge to the other person to prove the statement wrong. On the other hand, the group member could interpret the statement as criticism or confirmation of how things really are. The therapist must observe the reaction of the group members to each other's communication and be prepared to clarify, encourage, or interpret the meaning of the reaction and what was said.

Restore Cognitive Functioning. The assessment of self-understanding is essential to crisis resolution in group. Again, the therapist must attempt to motivate the group members to do the assessment but must clarify any inaccuracies and detrimental statements. The therapist should pay close attention to the group members' clarifications of another member's problems and functions because it will primarily be a projection of the member's feelings, and can provide helpful feedback about his or her own functioning.

Plan and Implement Treatment. Treatment actually began in the first interview and the first group session. At the conclusion of the first group session, however, the therapist should explain what will take place in the following sessions. In subsequent sessions the group should focus on problem solving and reinforcement of positive efforts. The therapist should encourage the group to evaluate efforts to change and improve coping methods. In any areas where improvement has not occurred, supportive understanding of why it has not occurred should also be a focus. The group must project an attitude of improvement and a concerted effort to feel, think, and behave more effectively. This must come about by a re-definition of the perceived meaning of the problem. So, in addition to self-understanding, there should be group effort to change perception and interpretation of the precipitating events and resultant situations. Alternatives to consequences caused by the precipitating event should also be a major focus. The therapist must discourage any group discussion that does not help any or all of the group members. When a group member has made sufficient progress, termination is indicated.

Terminate. Termination is indicated when the crisis has been resolved and the group member expresses confidence that he or she has improved the ability to function. Such a change can usually be determined by a change in feelings, perception, thinking patterns, and coping methods.

Follow-up. After a period of time, usually about six weeks, some contact with the client should be made to determine how well the client is doing. Follow-up not only offers support but also serves as an evaluation of the effectiveness of the treatment.

REFERENCES

Burgess, A. W. & Baldwin, B. A (1981) *Crisis intervention theory and practice. A clinical handbook.* Englewood Cliffs, N.J.: Prentice-Hall.

Comstock, B. & McDermott, M. (1975). Group therapy for patients who attempt suicide. *International Journal of Group Psychotherapy, 25,* (1), 44–49.

Erikson, E. H. (1959). Growth and crisis of the health personality. In Identity and the life cycle: Selected papers. [Monograph]. *Psychological Issues, 1* (1) 50–100.

Erikson, E. H. (1963). *Childhood and society.* New York: W. W. Norton.

Hartmann, H. (1958). Ego psychology and the problem of adaptation. [Monograph Series, No. 1]. *Journal of the American Psychoanalytical Association.*

Kalis, B. L., Harris, R. M., Prestwood, R., & Freeman, E. H. (1961). Precipitating stress as a focus in psychotherapy. *Archives of Generaly Psychiatry, 5*(3), 27–34.

Levy, R. (1982). *The new language of psychiatry: Learning and using DSM-III.* Boston: Little, Brown.

Lewis, A. B., Jr. (1973). Brief psychotherapy in the hospital setting: Techniques and goals. *Psychiatric Quarterly, 47*(3), 341–352.

Levine, B. (1979). *Group psychotherapy: Practice and development.* Englewood Cliffs, N.J.: Prentice-Hall.

McGuire, M. T. (1965). The process of short-term insight psychotherapy. II. Content, expectation and structure. *Journal of Nervous and Mental Disorders, 141,* 219–230.

Menninger, K., with Mayman, M., & Pryser, P. (1963). *The vital balance: The life process in mental health and illness.* New York: Viking Press.

Motto, J. (1979). Starting a theory group in a suicide prevention and crisis center. *Suicide and Life Threatening Behavior, 9,* (1).

Rapoport, L. (1970). Crisis intervention as a model of brief treatment. In R. W. Roberts & R. H. Nee (Eds.), *Theories of social casework,* pp. 267–311. Chicago: The University of Chicago Press.

Satterfield, W. (1977). Short-term group therapy for people in crisis. *Hospital and Community Psychiatry, 28,* (7), 539–541.

Strubler, M. & Allgeyer, J. (1967). The crisis group: A new application of crisis theory. *Social Work, 12* (3), 28–32.

Walker, W. J. (1953). Neurocirculatory asthenia. In F. C. Massey (Ed.), *Clinical cardiology.* Baltimore: Williams & Wilkins.

Yalom, I. D. (1975). The theory and practice of group psychotherapy. New York: Basic Books.

Yalom, I. D. (1985). The theory and practice of group psychotherapy. (3rd ed.) New York: Basic Books.

SUGGESTED READINGS

Kalis, B. L., Harris, R. M., Prestwood, A. R., & Freeman, E. H. (1961). Precipitating stress as a focus in psychotherapy. *Archives of General Psychiatry, 5*(3), 27–34.

Paul, L. (1966). Treatment techniques in a walk-in clinic. *Hospital and Community Psychiatry, 17*(2), 49–51.

6

Common Crisis Reactions

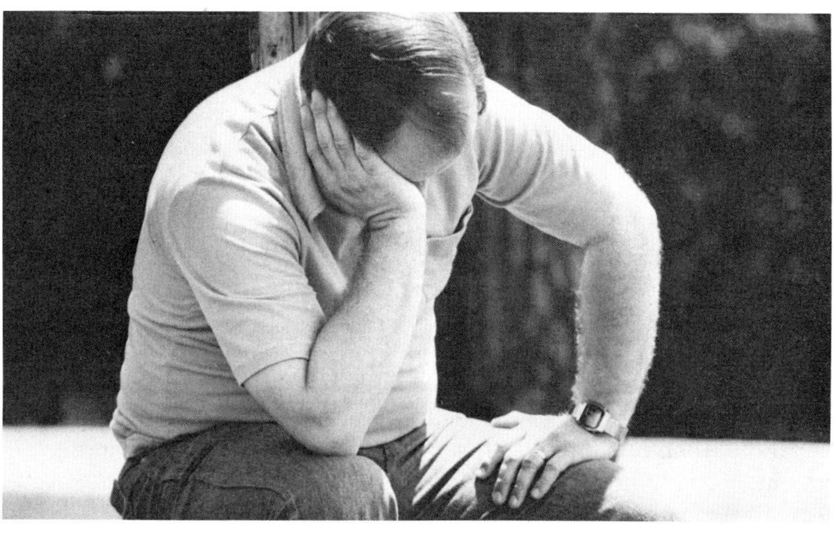

This chapter is designed to expand our knowledge and understanding of common crisis reactions and to make some suggestions for treatment. We have seen that it is the reaction to an event that causes a crisis, not the event itself. Consequently, effective crisis treatment requires treatment of the *reaction,* because the reaction is really the cause of the debilitation. Remember that once a person is unable to resolve a problem by usual methods and coping mechanisms, the emotional pain is overwhelming. As far as the person is concerned, the goal now is to alleviate this pain; solving the problem situation is abandoned. For example, if a husband's crisis is precipitated by his wife leaving him, he is usually not interested at first in why he is reacting in that way or what it means to him to be dependent on his wife. He is interested only in what to do to get his wife back so that his pain will be relieved and he can return to his precrisis status. Of course, his wife is a critical part of that. It follows, therefore, that the goal of the therapist is to alleviate the client's pain by doing whatever is necessary. The therapist may need to help get the wife back or may need to help the client see the difference between objective reality and his inner feelings that make it seem that he cannot live without her. The point is that the painful emotion is the cause of the debilitation. Thus it must be treated first. The first of the common emotional reactions that we will discuss is anxiety.

ANXIETY

Anxiety is a spontaneous response that acts as an alarm system, preparing an individual to defend against a potential danger. Anxiety developes whenever a person feels a threat to existence or to the values perceived to be necessary for existence; it will develop whenever someone feels that life or life-sustaining values or personality integration are threatened.

Anxiety, regardless of how irrational it is, can be the most painful of all human experiences. Its pain is intensified because its source is generally unknown. Furthermore, the human body cannot tolerate anxiety indefinitely. Prolonged anxiety must be alleviated by some psychological mechanism or it turns into a psychosomatic ailment. Laughlin (1967) reports the following case of death from panic anxiety:

> A 54-year-old man was admitted to the hospital because of marked anxiety accompanied by depression. He did not respond to treatment, and the anxiety increased. Rapidly he became severely anxious and agitated. Sedatives seemed powerless. He was apprehensive of death and he presented a clinical picture of the most acute anxiety. This unfortunate state continued unabated for well in excess of 48 hours, when he suddenly collapsed and died. The immediate cause of death was on postmortem examination reported to be "coronary insufficiency," accompanied by massive pulmonary edema. Pathologically, however, his coronary arteries were otherwise excellent. It was also difficult to explain the massive edema from any strictly pragmatic viewpoint. Seemingly, this patient had tolerated all of the acute anxiety of which he was physically, physiologically, and psychologically capable, and then death had supervened.

This case illustrates the importance of anxiety to psychic functioning. However, it is not the mere existence of anxiety that is a problem (as we saw in chapter 2), since a certain level of anxiety can be constructive and motivating. It is only excessive anxiety that is debilitating, and that is what we are concerned with here. When a crisis is manifested by overwhelming or excessive anxiety, the meaning is always the same: the individual feels relatively helpless to cope with a perceived danger to survival. He or she is, simply speaking, "scared to death." In using the word *anxiety* we imply that the cause of the reaction is subjective; there is no objective threat to survival. If there is an objective threat that is real in fact, we call the reaction *fear.* Thus cognitive restoration takes the form of reconciling the person's internal reality with objective reality.

There are three basic situations when a crisis is manifested by anxiety; that is, when the individual subjectively feels that (a) life is threatened, (b) control of a sexual or aggressive impulse is about to be lost, or (c) body integrity is perceived to be threatened.

Anxiety may arise when a person feels that life is threatened. This also includes the loss or threatened loss of a loved one who is perceived as necessary for survival (e.g., children who need parents for survival). It may also include the need for love.

Reacting to loss of a love object with anxiety differs from reacting with depression. If one reacts with anxiety, the meaning of the loss involves survival needs; if one reacts with depression, the meaning of the loss involves the need for love and self-esteem.

Anxiety may arise when an individual feels the imminent loss of sexual or aggressive impulse control. In such situations the usual methods of impulse control are progressively more ineffective, and anxiety develops to warn the person to do something quickly. Again, the threat of loss of impulse control is most often an unconscious cause of the anxiety, although some people can verbalize it. Verbalization is a good sign because conscious steps to avoid the loss of control can be taken. Two common examples of a fear of loss of impulse control are parents who develop anxiety over hurting their child and people in a homosexual panic. Consider the following case:

Mrs. Applebaum called the crisis center asking that her 3-year-old son be placed in a foster home. Mrs. Applebaum was obviously upset and crying profusely. After considerable difficulty she said that the reason she wants to put her son in a foster home is because he has been crying all day and she is afraid she may harm him. Discussion of the precipitating event revealed that the night before, she had gone out with friends and her ex-husband took care of their son. After she returned, he made a disrespectful comment regarding her "running around." She became so angry she broke a window. She was unable to sleep all night, and her son's crying all day was too much for her to handle.

Mrs. Applebaum had enough cognitive functioning to take preventive steps. Although she could verbalize that she was afraid that she would harm her son, she did not.

A fear of losing control of impulses that the person finds unacceptable or repugnant can sometimes result in depression rather than anxiety. At these times the conscience is operable in psychic functioning, in effect punishing the person for desiring the unacceptable. The notion of lust is an example.

Anxiety can reach crisis proportions when body integrity is perceived to be threatened. Recall that a negative reaction to forthcoming surgery is fear and not anxiety, because there is probably some danger inherent in all surgery requiring anesthesia.

The following two cases illustrate crises manifested by anxiety.

John, a 55-year-old accountant, requested an emergency appointment because his "nervousness" was affecting his performance on the job. When he was seen a few hours later, he appeared tense and restless; he was trembling. He said he did not know what was wrong with him. He had vague feelings of uncertainty and said there were times his legs felt so "rubbery" he thought he was going to fall to the ground. He was having difficulty sleeping and had begun to lose weight because of loss of appetite. When asked to describe how he felt, he related feelings of uneasiness, tenseness, anxiousness, and nervousness. John related his condition (precipitating event) to the sudden and unexpected notice that he was going to be transferred to his company's office in Arizona. He had been with the company in the same city for 24 years and had achieved the successful position of chief accountant. In the new position he would be the only accountant, performing the same duties as a beginner. In addition, a younger man was going to take John's position. All of this made John feel that he was being pushed out. This sudden and unexpected loss of position after 24 years, coupled with his considerable ego investment in the job and company, caused John substantial insecurity and tension. He did not know what to do. It all came so fast, so unexpectedly.

Brooke, a 29-year-old man, called the emergency services expressing a desperate need to talk to someone. He appeared anxious, red faced, and drained. The precipitating event causing his condition had occurred two nights before when his wife had told him that their marriage was over, that it was a mistake, and that she was bad for him. She then took off her wedding rings. Although they had only been married for a year, they had had a series of serious problems: his wife's hysterectomy, a step-daughter's operation for curvature of the spine, and the loss of his job, although he had since gotten another one. The wife's leaving was the last straw. Brooke expressed feelings of shakiness and an inability to sleep caused by his desperate need to be with his wife. He believed that if he could talk to her they could correct the situation, but she refused to talk with him. Brooke was sent home from work because his supervisor noticed his trembling and poor concentration. He believed that Brooke was too upset to work around machinery. It was at this time that Brooke called the emergency services.

Both John and Brooke reacted to their precipitating events with anxiety. John, for example, described feelings of nervousness, tenseness, restlessness, tremors, uncertainty, weakness in the lower extremities, loss of appetite, and sleeping difficulties, all characteristic of anxiety.

Reacting this way meant that John basically perceived the event as a threat to his survival. It is understandable why John would react with anxiety. He could feel that his transfer was the first step toward being fired and that after 24 years with one company he might not be able to get another job. Just as we can wonder why John reacted with anxiety, he probably also searched his mind for possible meanings of the precipitating event. This search can become the heart of the problem for the person in crisis. As the person searches his or her mind, imagination may take over. The person projects fears onto reality and reacts to them accordingly, often increasing the degree of anxiety and debilitation.

We treat the individual who reacts to a precipitating event with anxiety with the same nine steps discussed in chapter 5. The therapist can and should be more psychologically supportive in treating anxiety than depression. In anxiety, the person feels helpless, weak, and not confident. He or she feels scared and does not know what to do. The person cannot remember usual strengths and capacities. The therapist in such cases can actively encourage the client and reaffirm strengths. The therapist can help provide the client with hope and self-confidence again.

While the therapist is eliciting and encouraging the expression of painful feelings and emotions, focus should be on the physical symptoms, including a description of the physical sensation. If the client has chest pains or stomach pains, the therapist should ask the client to describe the feelings. (We are assuming that there are no organic causes for the client's physical symptoms. In such cases the therapist may want to inquire about the client's state of health or the last time he or she has seen a doctor.) If the individual simply says, "I feel anxious" or "I feel tense" or "I feel uneasy," the therapist should try to localize the feeling by asking, "Where do you feel tense?" or "Where do you feel uneasy?" This focus is therapeutic; it makes the client feel better because the therapist shows an interest in what the client is most concerned about now: the physical symptoms. It also satisfies the client's dependency needs and gives reassurance that help is available.

Having the client describe and discuss physical sensations can often be important in assesment and evaluation also. The physiological symptoms may at times be significant. For example, stomach pains can represent a perceived danger to dependency feelings; heart palpitations can represent guilt and anticipation of punishment (e.g., heart attack, death). Headaches can represent unexpressed anger and tension. Back pains and weakness in the legs can represent a desire to be dependent and to be completely helpless, confined to home or even to bed. The therapist should determine whether the anxiety symptoms are habitually expressed through the same physical system. If so, they are more likely to have idiosyncratic psychic meaning and value. Anxiety that is diffuse and manifested in several systems is less likely to have idiosyncratic meaning.

Another therapeutic value of focusing on the sensations of anxiety is the cognitive benefit. It forces the client to identify the pain, which helps to reduce the effects of feeling that the source of pain is unknown. At the same time, it tends to make the client aware that what is being experienced is anxiety. As the individual's anxiety decreases, the therapist moves to discussing the precipitating event and gathering information for the other therapeutic tasks (i.e., assessment and evaluation, identifying the nuclear problem, cognitive restoration, treatment planning, and implementation).

During cognitive restoration it is effective to explain the meaning of anxiety in words the client can understand (see step 6 in chapter 5). The client should understand that these feelings called "nerves" are anxiety. The client should immediately recall what anxiety means and search internally and externally for the cause. The client should compare what is in the mind with what is in the outside reality. In cognitive restoration, the relationship of the precipitating event to the crisis response should be clearly made.

Individuals vary in their ability to tolerate anxiety. However, those whose anxiety is overwhelming generally respond to steps we have discussed, especially to the therapist's encouragement to ventilate. Consider for example, the case of Vernon, who experienced homosexual panic.

Vernon, a 35-year-old professional man, called the crisis therapist requesting an immediate appointment. He started the session by saying that he was worried about his masculinity. He had recently developed thoughts that other men were thinking that he was "queer." As a consequence, he had to be careful that his behavior was not open to suspicion, that he could not notice another man scratch himself or pull up his trousers as they slipped down, for fear that they would wonder about him. He said that he was not worried about being a homosexual but was a little concerned about becoming one.

The therapist encouraged Vernon to express his feelings and concerns. After exploring the client's feelings, the therapist asked about the circumstances in which Vernon's panicky feelings were heightened. As expected, it happened when he was with a group of men, as his job required. He was still able to function, however, but had become increasingly worried that one of the men would notice and would see that Vernon was worried about his masculinity. The therapist used cognitive restoration to help Vernon recognize that he was attributing to others what was in his own mind and not real in fact; that he was reacting as if what was in his mind were real. Vernon's insecurity regarding his masculinity had started several weeks before when his wife left him. As the precipitating event, this was related to his condition, which was further reinforced by the nature of his job The therapist suggested that his wife's leaving undermined his confidence and his masculine self-concept. Since he said that he had never had any homosexual experiences, the problem was one of impulse control. This was stated to him in terms that he could understand. The therapist offered to refer him to a physician who could prescribe medication that could help him with his control problem. Vernon said that the session was very helpful and that he felt he was in control again. Another session was scheduled for the next day, one three days later, and one each for the next three successive weeks. Persons in homosexual panic should be seen frequently until the panic subsides, and they generally respond to a crisis model. However, two conditions should be considered in treating such individuals: (a) they are capable of being reactivated, and (b) in some, homosexual panic is the beginning of a schizophrenic process.

If anxiety is so overwhelming that all the therapeutic procedures, including ventilation, do not reduce its debilitating effects, referral to a physician for an antianxiety drug may be necessary. Other times, environmental modification may be necessary. One example is to place the client in a controlled environment that may reestablish feelings of safety and security. Final treatment planning should be based on the client's response to the therapeutic intervention, including the treatment planning and restoration. If there is sufficient reduction in anxiety, and cognitive functioning is restored, the client can continue to be treated in crisis therapy.

DEPRESSION

As discussed in chapter 2, people whose crisis is manifested by depression suffer from an overwhelming mood disturbance. Feelings such as dejection, sadness, despair, and self-depreciation are debilitating. Events that can precipitate a depression of crisis proportions are innumerable. However, there are four basic causes of debilitating depression: (a) loss or threatened loss of a love object; (b) loss or threatened loss of self-esteem, self-concept, or other ego values needed for psychic equilibrium; (c) failure to live up to internalized standards, expectations, values, or goals; and (d) violation or wish to violate some significant moral code or dictate. At the same time that the depressed person withdraws from people, he or she wishes for contact and gratification, often making repetitive complaints that help keep contact with others. The capacity to evoke in others a desire to help is both a danger and an aid. It is a danger in that gratification and attention from others are pitted against the internal feelings of unworthiness and guilt. In other words, the depressed person attempts to alleviate the pains of negative internal feelings of unworthiness by soliciting or demanding support and praise from others. The stronger the negative internal feelings, the greater the demands for attention from others. At the same time, the need for others renders the depressed person amenable to help. This dynamic understanding of the depressed should be the basis of treatment.

Treatment

In treating a depressed individual, the therapist should proceed with caution, at least until a constructive relationship has been established. Once, in an effort to support a depressed client, a therapist said, "Well, at least you're trying to do something about your situation by coming here." The client responded, "Even a dog will obey most of the time." This client was too severely depressed and lacking in self-esteem to accept support. The therapist should try to gauge the effects of intervention, particularly with severely depressed individuals. In such cases, dramatic improvement without corresponding time and effort could be a warning sign of suicide. It usually does not take very long to establish a constructive relationship with a client who is not severely depressed. The individual will throw out feelers very early on the qualities in the therapist to which he or she wants to relate. For example, about five minutes into the session, another depressed client said, "I went to the emergency room of Morton Hospital, and the guy they assigned to me was a trip; if I wasn't crazy when I went to him, I would have been when he finished with me." Although the therapist did not discuss this comment with the client, it raised questions as to the type of person the client wanted to relate to. To know what the client wants, the therapist simply needs to listen and hear what is being communicated. Until the therapist understands the depressed client, including what the client expects to get from the therapist, how the client uses interpersonal relationships, the client's need for punishment and degree of masochism, the therapist should not actively give psychological support. The natural response to seeing depression is to use psychological supportive techniques such as reassurance or praise to negate the client's feelings of hopelessness, self-depreciation, guilt, or inferiority, but initially a constructive relationship is inherently supportive enough. The therapist's genuine interest, respect, empathy, and desire to help the client will come across to the client. Additional active psychological support should be used sparingly and only when the client needs it and is willing to accept it as a source of hope and motivation.

A therapist at this point should be concerned with eliciting and exploring feelings, especially physical complaints. The therapist should inquire into the daily activities of the client. A very beneficial process with the depressed is to explore historical material to ascertain experiences and feelings of past interpersonal relationships, moving from spouse or loved ones to parents, siblings, and friends. This process helps the establishment of a constructive relationship, since it gratifies the client's dependency needs. Further, it facilitates the therapist's development of empathy and empathic understanding. This process is more than beneficial for the client; it helps the therapist to understand the client's psychic makeup and functioning. Furthermore, this focus interrupts the client's feelings of hopelessness and despair. Often the client will smile as he or she talks of past happy experiences or relationships. The therapist should not be overly concerned about the depressed client's dependency needs since this is a positive way to establish a constructive relationship rapidly. More important, it makes the client feel that relating to the therapist is going to be beneficial. Such a relationship not only gives the cognitive restoration process more impact, but it serves the function of reducing dependency after needs have been gratified appropriately.

Some depressed people will not be aware that they are depressed. They may feel "sad," "blue," or "down." In such cases it is therapeutic to suggest to the client that this is depression. For example, the individual who talks about constant fatigue, loss of interest in activities, and depletion of energy can be told gently that it sounds as though he or she is depressed. A frequent response is, "I've never thought of it that way." Sometimes a depressed client will feel that the therapist does not understand the seriousness of the condition. Sometimes if the client verbalizes such feelings to the therapist, the comments are designed to solicit sympathy or to make the therapist worry or feel guilty. The therapist who truly understands need not be manipulated by such an effort. Rather, the therapist can reassure the client of understanding and can express the hope of helping the client overcome depression.

Another factor in treating the depressed is that they are generally not aware of intense anger. Of course, the depression is caused by the fact that they have turned their anger inward. This is not to suggest that clients be encouraged to express anger simply as a technique. Anger should unfold naturally in the treatment process. Depressed individuals tend to attribute to others what they feel about themselves. For example, one wife constantly talked about how dissatisfied her husband was with her. She spoke of how critical he was and how she was unable to please him. When pressed for specific examples of how he was dissatisfied with her, she said he did not notice when she had cleaned out his closet. When she demanded that he recognize her effort he said, "Having a clean closet is not that important to me." This comment, she said, proved that he was unsatisfied with her. Appropriate cognitive restoration can be used to help the client become aware of how he or she attributes feelings about self to others. A therapist should be wary of trying to talk a depressed person out of guilt feelings by logic. This whole process serves as self-punishment. After the client has indulged in self-punishment, the therapist can relate the need for self-punishment and self-depreciation to the anger turned into the self. Also, the therapist can discuss the individual's feelings about anger, helping the client to recognize why he or she cannot express anger outwardly. The therapist can then point out that the client will continue to feel depressed until the real source of the anger is expressed outwardly.

The therapist should observe carefully the individual's reaction to what is said and let that guide what will be pursued. In treating depression, the therapist must use any hope and positive feelings the client shows. The therapist must be careful that, if using positive past behavior or performance of the client, the client is ready to receive it. It is generally best if hope is oriented toward the future. For example, Vivian, a 32-year-old doctoral student, had written all but the last chapter of her dissertation but felt unable to complete it. She appeared hopeless and felt incompetent. Rather than refer to the fact that she had completed all but one chapter, the therapist could support her hope and future accomplishments. For example, the therapist at one point said, "When you receive your Ph.D., you may be able to get the job with the new presidential administration." This was an appropriate comment in Vivian's case because getting a job with the Department of Health, Education and Welfare was her career goal and the basis for aspiration for a doctorate.

Some suggestions have been offered here for treating the depressed. Closely related is the subject of suicide, which we will look at next as we turn to the subject of violence.

CRISIS REACTIONS WITH POTENTIAL FOR VIOLENCE

Regardless of the setting or training, anyone working as a crisis therapist is likely to have as a client someone who is threatening or has the potential to commit violence (suicide or homicide) or who is a victim of sexual assault.

Suicidal Behavior

Menninger states: "Once every minute or even more often someone in the United States either kills himself or tries to kill himself with conscious intent. Sixty or seventy times each day these attempts succeed. In many instances, they could have been prevented (Schneidman and Farberow, 1957)."

It has been thirty years since Dr. Menninger made this statement. Today, suicide is the tenth-leading cause of death in the United States. More than one million people each year engage in suicidal behavior, and twenty-five thousand to fifty thousand actually kill themselves (Winder, 1983; Allen, 1977). The increasing incidence of suicidal behavior raises the likelihood that every therapist will encounter a client who is suicidal.

Suicidal behavior is an anxiety-producing subject because it defies the human instinct to survive. While most people are trying to live longer, suicidal people are either thinking about, attempting to, or succeeding at killing themselves. Suicidal clients not only produce anxiety in a therapist, but also tend to make the therapist rather angry as well (Kohler and Stolland, 1964; Ansel and McGee, 1971). Therapists feel responsible for their clients, but the client's unpredictability causes the therapist to feel anxious, helpless, and angry. There is a general tendency among therapists to blame oneself if a client succeeds in the suicide attempt. Consequently, therapists are too eager to dispose of suicidal clients. In this section we will try to understand suicidal behavior.

Suicidal behavior is viewed in this textbook as a crisis reaction to a precipitating event. It includes suicidal thoughts, gestures, attempts, and actualities.

There is no universally accepted cause of suicidal behavior. Most authors believe that there are multiple causes—psychological, social, and biological. For our purposes, the causes of suicidal behavior can be classified into three groups: psychosocial, psychopathological, and biological.

Psychosocial Causes. Psychosocial causes are the major determiners of suicidal behavior. Specifically, such behavior is precipitated by the disappointment related to the loss of a love relationship, loss of self-esteem, or some other psychosocial needs perceived to be of life-or-death importance. Hawton and Cataton (1983) found in their study of 132 suicide attempters that 72 percent of the attempts were precipitated by loss or disappointments in love relationships such as marital and boyfriend-girlfriend relationships. This finding suggests that when a person engages in suicidal behavior as a crisis reaction to the loss of a love relationship, the meaning of the loved one is overdetermined—in other words, there is more than one meaning beyond the current feelings of love. This reaction is exceptional since not everyone resorts to suicidal behavior at the loss of a significant loved one. Draper (1976) and Schneidman (1984) believe that people who react with suicidal behavior to loss or disappointment in love relationships have experienced the loss of a significant loved one at a critical period in their development; the occurrence of another such event produces unbearable pain covered over during the development process. The inability to solve the problems of the current precipitating event causes regression and the reactivation of the pain produced by the loss of the original loved one. When the suicidal individual is either unable to get the current loved person to return or to find a substitute, suicidal behavior is an attempt to escape from the unbearable pain. Draper (1976, p. 71) states:

> The primary request of the suicidal patient is the anesthesia that is administered by restoration of the previous state of well being that is fulfilled by the love or fantasied love of the ONE. This ONE is likely, of course, to be a transference figure in a current life situation embroidered with all the transference hopes and love fulfillment of the infant's mother.

The importance of Draper and Schneidman's positions relates the significance of the therapeutic relationship in understanding and treating suicidal behavior. Draper (1976, p. 75) states that "the rapport must be restorative of the hope for the love of the ONE and as such, is especially meaningful to the patient."

Crisis therapists working with suicidal clients must recognize the importance of both past and present relationships. The therapist must help the client recognize the connection between past pain produced by loss and current pain produced by loss. Most important, after the crisis of the suicide attempt is over, referral for long-term therapy should be made.

Another contributing psychosocial cause of suicide is family history. A history of suicide in one's family predisposes one to consider it as a way of solving difficult problems. If one identified closely with the suicidal family member, one might attempt suicide. Strong guilt feelings, religiosity, negative self-concept, and extreme loneliness can all contribute to suicidal behavior. The crisis therapist should consider at length the individual's perception of the meaning and the purpose of his or her life. The answer should be ascertained to the question, "What in reality does the client have that makes life worth living, as defined by the client?" The therapist also needs to ask, "What can I help this client find in life that makes it worth living?"

Psychopathological Causes. Although suicidal behavior is a crisis reaction to a precipitating event, it has a high incidence as a secondary condition in some psychopathological conditions.

The incidence of suicide is high in patients suffering from major depression, especially unipolar and the depressed phase of bi-polar, and, to a lesser extent, in schizophrenics. Kaplan and Sadock (1985) state that 15 percent of completed suicides are found in the undiagnosed or diagnosis-unspecified category of psychiatric illness. Borderline personality disorders are also high risk for suicidal behavior and other self-damaging acts. The therapist must always carefully assess and evaluate for suicidal potential any individual with a psychopathological condition.

Biological Causes. Biological factors known to contribute to suicidal behavior are alcohol, drugs, physical illness, and organic brain damage. Organic brain damage increases depression and impairs judgment so accidental overdoses of medication are common (Soreff, 1981). Age and gender are also highly correlated with suicidal behavior. Women make more attempts; men more often complete the act. The incidence of suicide increases with age.

Assessing Suicidal Potential

Perhaps the greatest concern of the crisis therapist is assessing the degree of suicidal risk; that is, attempting to reasonably predict the likelihood that a particular person will take his or her own life. All suicidal behavior, regardless of apparent significance, should be taken seriously. In a study of people who actually committed suicide, Schneidman and Farberow (1957) found that three-fourths had previously threatened or attempted to take their own lives. Some communication of suicidal intent is almost always given. If a suicidal statement, either explicit or implicit, is made simply in the context of the interview, the therapist should evaluate it immediately. The assessment and evaluation of suicidal potential should take place within the context of the major precipitating events (e.g., pain and disappointment in love relationships). With this in mind, the therapist should be concerned with the conditions of establishing a therapeutic relationship. The therapist must have empathy for the pain the suicidal person experiences, regardless of the manifest behavior. This empathy must be communicated through the process of empathic understanding.

Empathic understanding is not necessarily anything the therapist does or says; it is primarily an affective communication process transmitted from therapist to client. It is a meeting of feelings. Within this context, the therapist should explore the suicidal behavior directly as it is brought up. If allusion to suicidal behavior does not immediately come up, the therapist should wait for an appropriate time to introduce it, for example, when the client is talking about feelings of hopelessness or whether life is worth living. The therapist should not worry about putting ideas into the client's head. However, failing to explore suicidal indication, gestures, or attempts may make the client feel as if he or she is not being taken seriously. Almost all people who consider any form of suicide are at some point ambivalent or do not want to take their own lives. In fact, the individual whose motivation for suicidal behavior is disappointment in a love relationship most assuredly does not. The therapist must take advantage of that ambivalence by helping clients understand why they are experiencing these feelings. Suicidal behavior is an attempt to communicate, and the communication contains a message telling us why they are distressed and what they want others to know through their behavior and what is needed to relieve their distress. This point is illustrated by the case of Rosemary (see chapter 2), who came to the crisis center because she found a note written by her husband implying that he was going to commit suicide. First of all, nobody believed him, and second, what he needed to relieve his distress was a divorce, which Rosemary refused to give him. It is when no one hears the suicidal cry that the individual feels forced to resort to suicide. He or she simply feels there is no hope left. As Farberow and Shneideman (1961) found, suicide attempts are a cry for help. The cry, however, has to be decoded and interpreted. Inquiry into its meaning is therapeutic and ego reinforcing. To recognize and evaluate suicidal potential, the therapist must ask probing questions. When thoughts and feelings are expressed, they are separated in the client's mind from the actions.

With the support of the therapist, talking about suicidal thoughts can reduce the individual's feelings of helplessness and despair. Perhaps the first questions would involve suicide plans. The therapist could ask, "Do you feel so hopeless that you have thoughts about how you would take your life?" The more specific the plans, the greater the danger. And the more lethal the method, the greater the danger. Dwelling on thoughts of suicide is more serious than having transitory thoughts. If the individual says something like, "I've thought about suicide, but I'm too scared," it can be a good sign. Another consideration is the client's residual interpersonal relationships with significant others. A client who is concerned about the negative effects his or her death would have on relatives is showing some positive signs. If the therapist feels that the client has invested enough time that the relationship is meaningful, it is a very good sign. These are advantages of rapidly establishing a positive relationship. The client who denies that he or she will commit suicide is usually being truthful and can temporarily be relied on. Physical signs such as insomnia, weight and appetite loss, constipation, and lack of sexual interest are important in the evaluation of suicide danger. The greater the self-depreciation, the greater the danger. Going into and recovering from episodes of depression are also danger points. Other danger signs are a family history of suicide, repeated attempts, financial worries, and a sudden change in a significant relationship such as divorce or separation. The risk of completed suicide has been found to be higher among men (Susser, 1968), although women make more attempts. Homosexuals are prone to be suicidal, especially when depressed. People who live alone are more likely to commit suicide. Regan and Small (1966) summarize clues to suicide as follows:

> Classically, the therapist has many descriptive clues which help him to decide how much suicidal protection should be provided. More severe depressions, characterized by self-depreciation, feeling of worthlessness and hopelessness, nihilistic delusions, persistent self-destructive thoughts (especially of an aggressive nature), early morning awakening, anorexia with marked weight loss, amenorrhea, loss of sexual desire, and history of previous suicidal attempts by the patient or his relatives, are major indications for instituting precautions to avoid self-harm.

The crisis therapist must alert relatives and responsible friends to the client's suicidal potential. They should share the responsibility of prevention. Sometimes this concern can reverse the whole process. If suicidal potential is so severe that hospitalization is warranted, the client should be told and the family should be involved. A suicidal client should never be left to go to the hospital alone. The client should be given a feeling of being protected.

If a low suicidal potential makes protective custody unnecessary, the therapist can return to the normal course of treatment. This course should be guided by the knowledge of the individual's problems in love relationships. The nature and meaning of relationships (i.e., feelings of guilt, anger, and loneliness) should be the major focus of discussion. The therapist's goal is to help the client recognize what needs the client wants satisfied, how and why they have been ineffectually met in the past, and how change can help the client effectively meet them in the future.

After crisis treatment, the therapist must decide whether the client should be referred for traditional psychotherapy. From the perspective that the origin of suicidal behavior occurred at some phase of development, most non-psychotic suicidal people should be referred for long-term psychotherapy.

According to Meyerson, Glick, and Kiev (1976), the risk of a person taking his or her own life can be determined by three factors: lethality, intentionality, and attitude. Lethality refers to the choice of method, circumstances, and how close the individual comes to death. A gun is more lethal than aspirin, for example. Intent is determined by motivation; that is, the communicative purpose of the suicidal behavior (i.e., revenge, control, etc.).

Attitude is manifested by how the person's ego reacts to the suicidal behavior. It is ego-alien if the person feels ashamed, sick, scared or uncomfortable. It is ego-syntonic if the suicidal behavior is acceptable or comforting. Certain demographic characteristics are associated with suicidal risk. A therapist may find it helpful to be familiar with these. Walker (1983) identifies them in Table 6.1.

TABLE 6.1 *Factors associated with increased risk of suicide in emergency mental health patients*

	Factor	*Relatively Increased Risk If*
Identification	Age	Elderly[3, 17]
	Sex	Male[3, 17]
	Race	White or American Indian[3, 17]
	Marital status	Unattached, especially if divorced, widowed, or separated[3, 17]
Chief Complaint	Suicide attempt	Present, especially if attempt had high probability of fatality[8, 18] or if a note was left[8]
	Suicide ideation	Present, especially if patient had a definite plan or if he has a feeling of uncontrollable impulse[7]
Presentation	Commitment evaluation	Present[19]
	Alone	Present[8]
Present History	Onset of Symptoms	Acute[20]
	Stress	High, especially if due to physical illness[8] or loss of loved one[15]
	Diagnosis	Depression, alcoholism, or schizophrenia[4, 5, 7]
	Social isolation	Present[8]
	Reaction of others to symptoms	Rejecting[20]
Past History	Suicide attempts	Present, especially if attempts had high probability of fatality[18]
	Psychiatric disorders	Depression, alcoholism, or schizophrenia[4, 5, 7]
Family History	Suicide by close relative	Present, especially if a parent[14]
	Death of parent early in patient's life	Present[11]
Social History	Religion	Patient uninvolved in religion[14]
	Ethnicity	Northern European or Japanese[12]
	Job changes	Within 6 months[15]

TABLE 6.1 *Continued*

	Factor	*Relatively Increased Risk If*
Physical/Mental Status Exam	Medical illness	Chronic life-threatening especially if painful and disabling[21]
	Wrist scars	Present, especially if not mentioned prior to exam[22]
	Hallucinations	Present, especially if command self-destruction[21]
	Delusions	Present, especially if persecutory of external control[21]
	Response to interview	No relaxation or decrease in symptoms, no feeling of communication[17]

Note. From *Psychiatric Emergencies, Intervention and Resolution* by J. Ingram Walker, 1982. Philadelphia: J. P. Lippincott. Reprinted by permission. Copyright 1983 by J. P. Lippincott.

A complete assessment of suicidal behavior should include the precipitating event, social history, client personality, and the prediction of suicidal potential.

Treatment of the Suicidal Person

Treatment of the suicidal person begins with the first contact between client and therapist. We have emphasized the emotional pain the suicidal person has experienced throughout life because of disappointment in love relationships (Schneidman, 1984). This makes the therapeutic relationship of the utmost importance. Following the exploration of feelings and affect and the precipitating event, assessment of lethality should be done. If the individual is highly lethal, or when suicide is secondary to a serious psychiatric illness, steps such as hospitalization or protective custody should be taken to protect the person from harming himself or herself.

Often, lethality can be reduced in situations where realistic hope of change can be accomplished. For example, the therapist might be able to effect change by contacting a spouse, an employer, or whomever might be involved in the precipitating event. In such cases, the therapist does everything possible to effect a change in the client's life. All possible options should be discussed.

The therapist should not become anxious over the client's expectations of miracles. Nor should the therapist be disappointed if the client responds with "yes, but" or "I can't do that" to suggestions—remember that the suicidal client is ambivalent about life. The point is that while solutions are being explored, the client's cognitive function is increasing, and the lethality is being reduced.

Homicidal Behavior

We will use the phrase *homicidal behavior* to mean potential for or threat to commit physical harm to another individual.

A client that presents a threat of homicide can be frightening for the therapist. At the same time, a therapeutic response requires a calm, confident therapist who can take charge of the situation. The therapist should keep in mind that a threat of violence is an indication that the individual is struggling against losing control of self and is very frightened. Sometimes this fear may be hidden by a preoccupation with aggression or with boisterousness. Any person or situation that immediately counteracts this fear of loss of control is reassuring. Our concern is with the individual who wants help because he or she is afraid of committing a violent act (e.g., "I'm afraid I'm going to kill my child" or "I'm afraid I'm going to hurt someone"). Just as we have seen with anxiety and depression, the potential for homicide is also a consequence of an inability to cope with a crisis.

Again, the first task in intervening with a person who is potentially violent is to establish a constructive relationship rapidly. If the individual is obviously upset and angry and the therapist knows how the client feels, the therapist can move to the precipitating event or causes of the condition. If the client does not show the obvious emotions normally associated with violence, present feelings should be explored before moving to the causes of the need for violence. If the client's emotions are not consistent with the thought of violence, he or she may be planning future action. Consequently, thoughts and feelings should be examined before moving to precipitating events. Finding causes is extremely important for ego building, cognitive restoration, understanding the client's psychic structure, and for determining the nuclear problem. For example, if the precipitating event or cause of the individual's need to resort to violence is infidelity, humiliation, or insult, it is clear that there are ego needs involving self-esteem and feelings of worth and value. This means that the client is a very sensitive person who feels inadequate or inferior and must protect against the pain of these feelings. When an incident occurs that breaks down defenses against these feelings, the basic reaction to feeling hurt is to hurt back. The therapist must keep this kind of sensitivity in mind while actively getting involved with the client.

In working with the potentially violent, the therapist must act decisively and often directly. The therapist must be in charge. To do so, the therapist must gather a great deal of information and evaluate quickly. The therapist cannot hesitate to ask specific questions regarding the client's violence potential and life experiences. It is the information gained from these questions that the therapist uses to assess the risk of violence. Furthermore, it opens up cognitive functioning, again suggesting the need to be aware of consequences, a search for alternatives, and the provision of hope.

Certain historical patterns and experiences are predictive clues to homicide. Some people who experience severe emotional deprivation and rejection in early childhood will resort to violence in a crisis situation (Menninger and Modlin, 1972). This is understandable in light of the emotional satisfaction necessary for adequate psychic development and control of impulses. At the same time, not all people who experience severe emotional deprivation have so little impulse control. If emotional deprivation is a factor in homicidal tendencies, it generally will have been reflected in previous homicidal acts. Thus, a history of homicidal behavior or past problems of impulse control are reliable predictions of future homicidal behavior. The exception, of course, is the overly controlled, inhibited, shy, or passive person whose excessive control breaks down under the impact of the crisis. If such a person seeks help just before defenses break, that person should be evaluated as at high risk, and caution should be taken. In such cases, however, the reason the person seeks help for a lifelong problem at this point is important to understanding the individual. Seeking help is generally a positive sign, unless the client is coming to the therapist simply to achieve some other goal, such as to get a spouse back. Hellman and Blackman (1966) found that people with a childhood history of enuresis, fire setting, and cruelty to animals are more likely to be homicidal risks.

As when assessing suicidal behavior, the first step in ascertaining potential for violence is to take all threats seriously. Second, a discussion of the client's plans for violence should be thoroughly discussed. The question should be formulated in terms of the future, such as, "Since you have not been able to think of any other way to feel better, have you thought about how you might hurt John?" This question also suggests the reason for the violence. It simply reflects the natural human tendency to want to hurt back when one has been hurt. Careful consideration should be given to the precipitating event or the cause of the violence. MacDonald (1967) found that the more illogical or unjustified the reason for the homicide threat, the greater the risk. Conversely the more logical and justified the reason for the threat, the less the risk. Also, the more diffuse the direction the homicidal impulse takes, the less the risk. When the threat is directed at a specific person or object, especially if specific plans have been made, the risk is greater. In cases where the homicidal threat is directed toward a specific person, the nature of the client's relationship with that person should be thoroughly explored. This helps the therapist understand the meaning of that person to the client, as well as the client's psychic functioning. When homicidal thoughts are directed toward a loved one, that person should be interviewed when possible. Menninger and Modlin (1972) suggest that often in such situations the loved one unconsciously encourages the client to act violently. Sometimes when problems involve loved ones, they can be worked out or resolved conjointly. When the situation can be improved by involving another person, be it a loved one, minister, or friend, that person should be brought in when it is therapeutic and in the best interest of the client.

Another factor that should be considered as the therapist actively gathers information for the evaluation is the client's capacity for having satisfying interpersonal relationships. How does the client relate to people? Does the client tend to have good feelings about people? Does the client appear to have a conscience or to feel remorse? Does the client feel bad about what he or she feels like doing? Specifically, how does the client relate to the therapist? Is the client superficial and mistrustful? Does the client have a close friend? Or is the client overly self-centered as a defense against feelings of inadequacy or inferiority? What is the client's relationship with members of the opposite sex? If the client is a man, does he unduly need women to sustain his ego and to meet dependency needs on the one hand, while being violently angry at them on the other? (This question applies to women also; however, more men than women become homicidal in reaction to disappointment in love relationships.)

Another consideration in evaluating homicidal potential is the client's culture. The client who is a member of a culture in which violence is considered acceptable is more likely to act out violently. Also, the client who is sociopathic is more likely to be homicidal. Obsessive homicidal thoughts are common in parents who fear that they are going to hurt their children. If these parents deny that they want to do so and appear to have good impulse control through defense mechanisms such as undoing (expiating guilt by symbolic acts), reaction formation, denial, or rituals or compulsive acts, the risk is less. However, if the immediate problem cannot be alleviated in the usual crisis time limit, referral to traditional therapy should follow.

In sum, a homicidal threat should be taken seriously. All of the clues suggested here should be explored as part of the assessment and evaluation process. Treatment then should be formulated and implemented accordingly.

Treatment

Treatment of the homicidal client follows the same procedures and steps as other crisis treatment. Cognitive restoration allows the client to understand the meaning of the behavior, separating thought from action. The therapist must appeal to the positive ego functions and strengths. Before seeking help, the client has been simply acting. The cognitive restoration process enables the client to think about these actions. Chances are the client will do that throughout the session, but at this point, with the help of the therapist, the client can cognitively relate behavior to thoughts about reasons and alternatives.

The first act of the treatment process is to decide, based on the assessment and evaluation, whether the client needs protective custody. Hospitalization or a halfway house of a mental health facility may be needed.

If the client needs hospitalization for self-protection, he or she should be informed and relatives should be notified and brought into the situation. They should assume responsibility for getting the client to the hospital if they can. Sometimes referral to a physician is necessary. If hospitalization is not necessary but some control is needed, the therapist can assess whether the family can provide the needed protection. Sometimes this can be combined with medication, in which case referral to a psychiatrist should be made. The therapist ensures as well as possible that the client will go to the psychiatrist.

At the conclusion of the session, the therapist may believe that the threat of homicide can be worked out by crisis therapy, and proceeds accordingly. However, the therapist should especially be concerned with helping the client ventilate as a means of reducing aggressive impulses. The therapist should help the client recognize the reason for the desperation and should work toward increasing the client's cognitive functioning, especially perception, judgment, and reality testing. When reality testing is poor, people are unable to recognize the consequences of their behavior. Environmental manipulation should be used to make the client's life less stressful. The therapist should consider interviewing the loved ones involved. Most violent acts are against loved ones and friends rather than strangers. Understanding the threat of violence towards loved ones can be very effective in preventing it. If removing the client from the environment is indicated, it should be recommended. For example, the therapist might recommend that a potentially brutal husband move in with friends for a few days while he works on his problem.

Sexual Assault

Sexual assault is the third form of violence to be discussed in this chapter. For our purposes, sexual assault is defined as an act of sexual intercourse between a male and a female, against her will, and under the threat of violence or physical harm. It is the fastest-rising violent crime in the United States (McCombie, Bassuk, Savitz, and Pell, 1976; Rada, 1978). Yet the victims of sexual assault are just now beginning to receive the attention they deserve from the community. This increased attention is due more to the women's movement than to the increase in incidence of the crime.

The victim of sexual assault needs the therapeutic help of a comprehensive support system more than the victims of other violent crimes do. Ideally, a crisis therapist should be a part of, or immediately available to, every hospital emergency room. One should be assigned to each police unit answering the call of rape. Consider the following case*:

> If I had to do it again, I would never have gone through with the prosecution. "I wouldn't even have reported it." said one twenty-seven-year-old woman who suffered through months of legal proceedings and publicity only to see her rapist found innocent because she was unable to prove that she did not consent to the act. Despite extensive body bruises and a wound in her forehead that took six stitches to close, the defense attorney argued that "vigorous love play" did not necessarily indicate nonconsent and, in fact, could even indicate enthusiastic approval and passionate involvement in the act.
>
> "From the beginning I had this feeling that I was the one who was on trial rather than the guy they picked up and charged." said the woman, raped by an intruder who entered her apartment through a window, from an adjacent rooftop. She was at the time sleeping in the nude, a fact that is frequently alleged in rape cases to prove "willingness to have intercourse."
>
> Right after it happened . . . I mean, here I was lying on the floor, my face was streaming with blood, I was damned near hysterical when I called the police. They arrived and the very first question this one guy asked me was, "Did you enjoy it?" "Did you really try to resist the guy?"
>
> Then the questions really started. I couldn't believe what they asked me. About five officers were crowded into my bedroom. They said things to me like "Lay on the bed exactly as you were when the guy came in. Why did you spread your legs if you didn't want to be raped? Did you see his penis? Describe it. Did you touch his penis? Did you put it in your mouth? Did you have an orgasm?"
>
> Then there was the hospital they took me to. There were maybe three dozen people sitting around in this large ward. This one guy in a white coat takes my name and he yells down the ward, at the top of his lungs,

---

*From *Sisters in Crime* by F. Adler, 1975, New York: McGraw-Hill. Copyright 1975 by McGraw-Hill Book Co. Reprinted by permission.

> "Hey, Pete, I got a rape case here. Check her out, will you?" It was just incredible. The guy checking me out left me sitting on this table for like an hour. One of his questions was, "Did you give the guy a blow job or what?"
>
> Later at the police station. They caught the guy from my description. He was sitting there, and one of the cops went out to get him a cup of coffee and gave him a cigarette. They told me, "Sit over there, lady, we'll get to you in a minute."
>
> Over and over again, the police, the district attorney, the defense attorneys, even my own goddamned private lawyer asked me the same thing: "Are you sure you really resisted? Did you really want to get raped subconsciously?"
>
> In the end the guy who did it got off. They even brought in this one boy—a man now—that I knew in high school. That was ten years ago. He testified he had intercourse with me, after a prom. The defense attorney said, "She was pretty easy, wasn't she?" The guy just grinned and shook his head.

Although there has been an increase in the number of sexual assault crisis centers, all victims do not go to these centers first, or even know they should go there. Access to needed services is determined by the community. A large percentage of sexual assaults still are not reported for various reasons, including feelings of guilt or shame or lack of knowledge. Greater sensitivity to the emotional and psychological effects on the victim must be developed by the support network, especially police and lawyers. Sexual assault is a reprehensible crime that not only violates the victim's human rights but can result in irreparable psychological damage, not to mention physical harm and even death. People in the helping network must be sensitive to this danger to prevent psychological damage and to reduce the victim's fear of reporting this hideous crime.

Some Characteristics of the Sexual Assault Victim

Burgess and Holmstrom (1974) found several physical and emotional characteristics generally manifested by the sexual assault victim. Physical symptoms resulting from trauma were soreness and bruises all over the body, especially on the legs, arms, chest, thighs, and neck. Physical symptoms also occurred in the area of the body that was the focus of attack. For example, victims who were forced to have oral sex reported irritation to the mouth and throat. Those forced to have vaginal and anal sex reported experiencing vaginal discharge, itching, burning sensations on urination, generalized pain, and rectal pain and bleeding. Tension headaches, sleep disturbances, stomach pains, appetite loss, and increased motor activity are also common manifestations.

Contrary to expectation, Burgess and Holmstrom (1974) did not find that shame and guilt were the primary reactions. Understandably it was fear of physical injury, mutilation, and death. The primary feeling of fear was also associated with a variety of other symptoms such as humiliation, shame, guilt, anger, and a desire for revenge.

Treatment

The first step in the treatment of the sexual assault victim is to establish a constructive relationship rapidly. This requires considerable sensitivity and empathic understanding. She may have a variety of ambivalent and confusing feelings including guilt, self-blame, shame, fear, anxiety, uncleanliness, and feelings of being damaged. Sensitivity is greatly facilitated by the therapist's perception of sexual assault as an act of violence with the potential of serious damage. Orzek (1983) believes that a female therapist is preferable because of a natural empathy and understanding; that a male therapist may deal with the sexual aspects of the sexual assault more than with the violence involved. It is possible for a male therapist to have the same degree (if it could be measured) of empathy as a female therapist; however, the fact that the client has been victimized by a man can pose some problems. One problem can be overreaction on the part of each: the male therapist becoming oversolicitous and the victim overly angry at the therapist simply for being a man. It is not always possible for the victim to be assigned to a female therapist. When a male therapist is assigned, he should be sensitive and aware of whatever feelings the victim has about seeing a man. He should explore her feelings early to help establish a constructive relationship.

The second step in working with the victim of sexual assault is dealing with the emotional reaction. As in every crisis, there is an initial state of upset. For the sexual assault victim, it is initially anxiety, fear, and shock, all contributing to psychic disequilibrium and a threat of personality disintegration. From our understanding of anxiety, we can see that the sexual assault victim is at first overwhelmed with fear for her bodily integrity and survival. During this phase the therapist works toward a complete expression of her painful feelings and emotions. While eliciting maximum ventilation of painful feelings, the therapist begins the third step by having the victim discuss the assault (the precipitating event) by discussing what happened, how, and the circumstances surrounding it. The therapist must understand the victim's total perspective of sexual assault. The therapist needs to know what happened to her. If there is any misinformation or erroneous sexual knowledge, it should come out as she talks about what happened. Thoroughly discussing the precipitating event—the sexual assault—is very important, regardless of how painful it is. It is a basic premise of crisis theory that to resolve the crisis successfully, the individual must face the precipitating event and thoroughly express her feelings about it, no matter how painful.

Discussing the assault lets the therapist and the client share the client's experiences. It is at this time that the circumstances surrounding the sexual assault are described. Information on the setting and how the act occurred is obtained to help in assessment of the problem. The victim should talk about any feelings of her own personal contribution, if any, to the assault in terms of acts omitted and committed. Was the victim unusually careless? Was she in a strange neighborhood at a time when she would be vulnerable? Did she take undue chances? It is not unusual for the victim to feel guilty and full of self-blame. The expression of these feelings should not be discouraged or negated by the therapist saying, "It was not your fault." Even though it was not her fault, if she feels a need to share such feelings, she should be allowed to do so. Usually the victim who feels responsible for the attack will voluntarily talk about these feelings. When this is not the case, the therapist can simply say, "Tell me what happened."If the victim does not want to discuss the horrible experience and says that she wants to forget it, she should be encouraged to discuss and face it, as she can never forget it. As emotions flow, the therapist must be supportive and empathic in the attempt to help the client sort out the differences between her feelings and reality. Universalization is used to support the victim's feelings and to let her know that she is not alone in her feelings; that it is natural for her to feel what she is feeling after being assaulted.

Step 4, the assessment phase, is modified somewhat for the victim of sexual assault. During this phase the therapist is most concerned with identifying the nuclear problem, which is the meaning of the sexual assault to the victim, rather than purely the causes of her reaction. We see that basically the sexual assault has two meanings, as the client moves from manifestations of anxiety to depression. Most sexual assault victims move from initially being overwhelmed with anxiety, that is, concern with bodily integrity and survival, to depression, or concern with feelings of loss, loss of a loved one, self-esteem, shame, and other interpersonal relationships. We want to understand what the event means to the victim and how she interperets the meaning to herself; that is, what does it mean to her now, and what will it mean in the future. The victim often degrades herself, which is characteristic of the depressed. The therapist should allow her to experience the pain of her own recriminations. The therapeutic task here is to share the victim's pain, understanding and accepting how she can feel the way she does. She needs to do this as a part of the restoration process. Part of this need for recrimination is due to the natural feelings that she could have done more to prevent it. Such feelings of self-blame are also characteristic of the depressed. We see such feelings in the bereaved and in people experiencing other kinds of personal losses. The other aspect of the assessment and evaluation phase is to determine whether the victim's responses are average and expectable or whether they indicate incipient psychosis or other clinical syndromes.

Step 5, formulating a dynamic explanation, involves reconciling the meaning of the event to the victim and the circumstances surrounding its occurrence. Here we are concerned with objectively understanding whether the victim contributed to the occurrence of the event by not taking "reasonable" precautions or whether it was impossible for her to prevent it. If the victim was careless and did not take all possible precautions, the therapist is interested in determining what this means to her psychic functioning. This is not because the therapist is any less sensitive or empathic. It is because the therapist wants to understand the psychic structure of the individual in crisis and what her behavior means to her overall psychic functioning and to her future social functioning. Such behavior may indicate the need for long-term psychotherapy.

The therapist should evaluate the victim's own supportive resources, especially loved ones, family, and close friends. This means that the therapist may need to help the victim resolve any reluctance to tell loved ones what happened. After discussing with the victim who she will tell, the decision needs to be made as to how this will be accomplished. The victim can decide to tell other people herself, the therapist can do it for her, or they can do it together. The victim's feelings regarding the loved ones' reactions will need to be handled and worked through if necessary. There are times when negative reactions of husbands or relatives will require therapeutic work for the victim's benefit.

The Male Partner

When a woman has been sexually assaulted, she feels reverberations in every aspect of her life, especially her relationship with her male partner. His reaction to this event is dependent upon the quality of the preexisting relationship and his beliefs concerning sexual assault (Orzek, 1985). If possible, the therapist should privately see the male partner of the victim. It would be best, when possible, that a male therapist see the male partner (Orzek, 1985). In working with the male partner, feelings about the assault should be explored. He should discuss the personal effect of the assault on both himself and his relationship with the victim. He should be encouraged to view the assault as an act of violence, not a sexual act (Burgess and Holmstrom, 1979). Identification with the victim should be fostered. If the relationship is secure and supportive, the trauma will be less severe.

It should be emphasized that step 6, cognitive restoration, is implemented only after lengthy and complete ventilation and expression of feelings and emotions. This phase for the sexual assault victim can take two directions. The first is to help the victim understand the meaning of her post-traumatic behavior. This is necessary to help her integrate the experience. The second direction is to help the victim cognitively accept the event. In these situations, cognitive restoration involves helping the victim accept the fact that there was nothing she could have done to prevent the event and to reconcile reality with her emotional feelings—her psychic reality. Inherent in both of these tasks is still the realization that a violent act has been committed and that, regardless of the circumstances, any person ought to be able to go anywhere he or she wants at any time and under any condition and not have his or her body violated. But such is not a fact of life. Additional treatment in this session should involve helping the client with practical arrangements.

Practical Arrangements

After the crisis has subsided and some cognitive functioning has been restored or improved, the therapist should help the victim with some necessary practical tasks to which she should attend. Although the therapist should encourage the victim to do everything she can for herself, the therapist should be there for support and encouragement, and to do those things that the victim cannot do herself. The first task is medical treatment. If the victim has not received medical treatment, the therapist should arrange for her to have a physical examination, including tests for venereal disease. Slaby and associates (1975) recommend several methods to prevent pregnancy. Such medical matters can be discussed with the victim's attending physician. A female physician is recommended when possible.

Another practical task that the therapist should help with is obtaining an attorney. This should be done whether the victim presses charges or not. In many cases the therapist will have to help the victim through ambivalent feelings about pressing charges. There are numerous reasons for such indecisiveness, including police procedures, which can be very dehumanizing. Fox and Scherl (1972) found that the greater the degree of self-blame, the less willing the victim was to report the crime.

Sometimes it is therapeutic for the sexual assault crisis therapist to accompany the victim to the medical facility and the police station. In any event, the victim should not be left to go to those places alone.

Perhaps the final practical arrangement is to help the victim deal with anticipated consequences of the assault. Court trials are notoriously brutalizing, and she will be subjected to a defense attorney who is trying to prove that no sexual assault occurred and who may resort to all types of dirty tricks. The victim should be aware of what she will have to go through. Other upsetting consequences include fear of returning to the same location or fear of another assault. Reasonable precautions that would alleviate these fears can be discussed. It is often therapeutic to suggest that the sexual assault victim not stay alone for a few nights, if she lives by herself.

Not all sexual assault victims need more than is discussed in the first session. However, the first session can take hours. After the anxiety over bodily integrity and survival have passed, the victim may again become depressed, and additional sessions will be required. Much of the anger at the attacker or at a nonaccepting judgmental husband or relative is turned inward. The victim may still feel guilty, unclean, or damaged. She will need help in working through these feelings. If they are too intense, too tenaciously held, and do not respond to usual therapeutic techniques, she may be showing signs that a clinical syndrome is developing. Further evidence of this would be reflected in her overall social functioning, her interpersonal relationships, functioning on her job, personal habits, and thought processes.

Just as with any other crisis condition, when the sexual assault victim is restored to her preassault level of social functioning, therapy can be terminated. Sometimes this occurs after the first session; other times it requires several sessions. If the victim does not return to her precrisis level of social functioning, she should be referred for traditional psychotherapy. The exception, of course, is if another precipitating event associated with the original assault occurs such as becoming pregnant or separating from her husband as a consequence of the assault.

BEREAVEMENT AND GRIEF

George died at age 55, swiftly and unexpectedly. Joanne, a professional nurse, appeared strong and unshaken as she dramatically carried out the practical arrangements of the funeral and greeting the many sympathizers and mourners. When a friend remarked about how well she had been holding up under the stress and strain, she said, "These tranquilizers are doing a great job. I have to be strong for the children. George would have wanted it that way." Several months after George's death Joanne came to the crisis center, saying that she could no longer go on living.

Joanne did not allow herself to experience the normal grieving process. She never got beyond the shock and denial phase and refused to emotionally accept her loved one's death.

Bereavement is the loss of a loved one through death, and grief is the emotional and behavioral reaction to the loss. Grief is a universal phenomenon. It is based on the inevitability of human mortality and the innate need of people to attach themselves first to parents and later to others. We will look further at why grief is such a painful but necessary process. Through introjection and identification, these attachments become an integral part of the psychic system. They are instrumental in social functioning, specifically in meeting emotional needs and maintaining psychic equilibrium and happiness. Therefore, when people lose a loved one, they in effect lose a part of themselves. Although there are normal characteristics of the grieving process (to be discussed later), specific patterns of reactions are influenced by three basic conditions. The first is the nature and meaning of the survivor's relationship to the deceased. This includes the ambivalent feelings inherent in every close or intimate relationship, including the love and hate, dependence and independence, repressed anger, and overdependency. The meaning of the relationship refers to the significance of the deceased to the psychic system and functioning of the survivor. The spouse who is overly dependent on the deceased will have, as a rule, a more difficult grieving process than those who are appropriately dependent.

The second condition is the degree of identification with the deceased. Identification is part of the love process, but in this case, identification with the deceased refers to the survivor's projection of self in the place of the deceased. Problems occur when there is overidentification, when the survivor sees self too much in the position of the deceased, preventing the appropriate management of the grief process and participation in the practical arrangements, a very important part of the grieving process. In fact, this is the purpose of funerals; they are for the benefit of the living. Consider the example of Fred, a 44-year-old, successful lawyer who could not visit his wife in the hospital while she lay terminally ill, let alone make funeral arrangements for her when she died. While all of this was going on, he disappeared for more than nine weeks, living the life of a recluse. He was drinking himself into oblivion until he was able to face the reality of the situation. Relatives and friends condemned Fred's behavior, since they were unable to understand or accept the way he handled his grief. Fred was not only unable to face his wife's death, he could not face her, since he overidentified with her. She reminded him of his own mortality.

Underidentification is more difficult to observe because of the social pressure and expectation to grieve. Furthermore, it can have many causes, including relief or even happiness that the "loved one" has died. In underidentification, the survivor is concerned with the benefits gained from the death of the deceased. Perhaps a common example is the terminally ill loved one who is conscious of impending death and lingers on and on, creating hardships for the survivors. Living with this kind of awareness is no doubt very painful for the terminally ill, but it is also painful for people who love him or her. They may become angry and wish the person would die quickly so they can "get back to normal." After the death they may feel guilty about those feelings.

The third condition is the age of the bereaved. The grieving process is generally more difficult for very young and elderly survivors. The reason, of course, is that young people and old people often are quite dependent on others. It is more difficult for them to adjust and fill the void. This is especially true of the elderly, who now must deal with fewer resources than they once had and fewer chances of developing new relationships to replace the old one.

Grief As a Normal Process

Some characteristics of a normal grieving process can be identified. Lindemann (1944) declares:

> The picture shown by persons in acute grief is remarkably uniform. Common to all is the following syndrome: sensations of somatic distress occurring in waves lasting twenty minutes to an hour at a time, a feeling of tightness in the throat, choking with shortness of breath, need for sighing, an empty feeling in the abdomen, lack of muscular power, and an intense subjective distress described as tension or mental pain.

Lindemann also adds as common characteristics a slight sense of reality, a feeling of increased emotional distance from other people (sometimes they appear shadowy or small), and intense preoccupation with the image of the deceased. If we examine these characteristics, it becomes clear that the grieving process involves emotional and behavioral manifestations of anxiety and depression (see chapter 2). Depression in grief is somewhat different than depression caused by other events. Guilt and anger may be present in grief, but less intensely. At one level, the grieved remains hopeful that the pain will eventually pass. Grief involves rational expression of feelings. A grieving person does not feel inferior or less of a person because of the loved one's death; self-esteem is not greatly altered. Crying spells are related to feelings about the deceased and preoccupation with self (e.g., "I don't know what I'm going to do"). The grieving person evokes sympathy but is often more concerned about the pain of others. It is not unusual for the grieving person to wish he had treated the deceased better or told him that he was loved and so forth.

It is not unusual for normal grief to last from six months to a year. Lindemann (1944) states that the length of the grieving process depends on how well the individual does the grief work; specifically, how well he or she emancipates himself or herself from the bondage to the deceased, readjusts to the environment in which the deceased is missing, and forms new relationships. Normal grieving is successful when there is emotional and psychological acceptance of the loss of the loved one, when there is a return to psychic equilibrium, when social functioning is directed once again toward personal goals and the persuit of happiness, and when memories can be recalled without pain, but with joy, pride, or pleasure.

Grief As a Crisis Condition

Grief reaction is a crisis when the deceased is so significant to the survivor that the loss is overwhelming and causes overall social dysfunctioning and emotional debilitation. It may become a crisis if the nature of the relationship between the survivor and the deceased was one of ambivalence and unacceptable hostility on the one hand, and guilt on the other. It becomes a crisis when the death of the loved one cannot be emotionally accepted. It becomes a crisis when painful feelings of sorrow, hurt, and loneliness cannot be adequately expressed.

Treatment of Grief As a Crisis Condition

The treatment of grief as a crisis condition follows the basic steps set forth in chapter 5. Most important are eliciting and encouraging the expression of painful feelings, including crying. Tranquilizers should not be used unless necessary, since they prevent the maximum expression of feelings. No feelings should be discouraged, not even idealized ones or the need to review the past. The bereaved should be helped to remove the obstacles to natural grief work such as use of denial or immediate involvement in another love relationship. The client must be helped to do grief work and encouraged to express feelings and emotions. The client should be allowed to talk about the deceased in whatever way he or she wants. Expression of feelings and emotions may take two to three sessions before the dynamic formulation and cognitive restoration phase. The dynamic formulation involves determining the reason for overreaction. The answer can generally be found in one of the three conditions discussed earlier: the nature and meaning of the relationship, the degree of identification, or the phase of the life cycle. The use of cognitive restoration may have to be delayed until later sessions. It is determined by the bereaved's readiness for emotional lifting. The therapist may encourage and motivate the bereaved to get back into normal social relationships. Some direct advice and prescription of what to do may have to be offered. If the client offers resistance to recovery, it has to be handled. The therapist should be alert to the expression of any suicidal ideation or bizarre behavior. The distinction between depression proper and grief work should be observed. Family and relatives should be used as resources when indicated. Termination can occur when there is an emotional acceptance of the loss and restoration of psychic equilibrium and adequate social functioning.

In this chapter we have discussed some common reactions of the individual in crisis. As we move to the next chapter, more than one individual in crisis will be discussed, namely, the family in crisis. We will also discuss three major crisis conditions associated with the task of the life cycle, specifically adolescence, middle age, and old age.

REFERENCES

Adler, F. (1975). *Sisters in crime.* New York: McGraw-Hill.

Allen, N. (1977). History and background of suicidology. In Hatton, C., Valente, S., & Rink, A. *Suicide: Assessment and intervention.* New York: Appleton-Century-Crofts.

Ansel, E., & McGee, R. (1971). Attitudes toward suicide attempters. *Bulletin of Sociology, 8,* (69).

Burgess, A. W., & Holmstrom, L. L. (1979). Sexual assault, sexual disruption and recovery. *American Journal of Orthopsychiatry, 49* (4) 648–657.

Burgess, A. W., & Holmstrom, L. L. (1974). *Rape: Victims of crisis.* Bowie, Md.: Robert J. Brady.

Draper, E. (1976). A developmental theory of suicide. *Comprehensive Psychiatry, 17* (1).

Farberow, N. L., & Shneidman, E. S. (1961). *The cry for help.* New York: McGraw-Hill.

Fox, S. S., & Scherl, D. J. (1972). Crisis intervention with victims of rape. *Social Work, 17,* 37–42.

Hawton, K., & Cataton, J. (1982). *Attempted suicide: A practical guide to its nature and management.* New York: Oxford University Press.

Hellman, D. S., & Blackman, N. (1966). Enuresis, fire-setting and cruelty to animals: A triad predictive of adult crime. *American Journal of Psychiatry, 122,* 1431.

Hoffman, D. L., & Remmel, M. L. (1975). Uncovering the precipitant in crisis intervention. *Social Casework, 56,* 259–267.

Kaplan, H. I., & Sadock, B. J. (Eds.). (1985). *Comprehensive textbook of psychiatry* (Vols. 1 and 2). (4th ed.).

Kohler, A., & Stotland, E. (1964). *The end of hope.* London: Collier-Macmillan.

Laughlin, P. (1967). *The neuroses.* Reading, Mass.: Butterworths.

Lindemann, E. (1965). Symptomatology and management of acute grief. In H. J. Parad (Ed.), *Crisis intervention: Selected readings* (pp. 7–21). New York: Family Service Association of America. (Reprinted from *American Journal of Psychiatry,* 1944, *101*).

MacDonald, J. M. (1967). Homicidal threats. *American Journal of Psychiatry, 124*(4), 475–482.

McCombie, S. L., Bassuk, E., Savitz, R., & Pell, S. (1976). Development of a medical center rape crisis intervention program. *American Journal of Psychiatry, 133*(4), 418–421.

Menninger, R. W., and Modlin, H. C. (1972). Individual violence: Prevention in the violence-threatening patient. In J. Fawcett (Ed.), *Dynamics of violence.* Chicago: American Medical Association.

Meyerson, A. T., Glick, R. A., & Kiev, A. (Eds.). (1976). *Psychiatric emergencies.* New York: Grune and Stratton.

Orzek, A. (1983). Sexual assault: The female victim, her male partner and their relationship. *Personnel and Guidance Journal, 62* (3), 143–146.

Rada, R. T. (Ed.). (1978). *Clinical aspects of the rapist.* New York: Grune & Stratton.

Regan, P. F., & Small, S. M. (1966). Brief psychotherapy of depression. In J. H. Masserman (Ed.) *Current psychiatric therapies* (Vol. 6). New York: Grune & Stratton.

Shneidman, E. S. (1984). Aphorisims of suicide and some implications for psychotherapy. *American Journal of Psychotherapy, 38,* (3).

Shneidman, E., & Farberow, N. L. (Eds.). (1957). *Clues to suicide.* New York: McGraw-Hill.

Slaby, A. E., Lieb, J., & Tancredi, L. P. (1975). *Handbook of psychiatric emergencies.* Flushing, N.Y.: Medical Examination Publishing.

Soreff, S. M. (1981). *Management of the psychiatric emergency.* New York: John Wiley & Sons.

Susser, M. (1968). *Community psychiatry: Epidemiologic and social themes.* New York: Random House.

Walker, J. I. (1983). *Psychiatric emergencies intervention and resolution.* Philadelphia: J. P. Lippincott.

SUGGESTED READINGS

Bach-y-Rita, G., Lion, J. R., Ailment, C. E., & Ervin, F. R. (1971). Episodic dyscontrol: A study of 130 violent patients. *American Journal of Psychiatry, 127,* 1473–1478.

Burgess, A. W., & Holmstrom, L. L. (1974). *Rape: Victims of crisis.* Bowie, Md.: Robert J. Brady.

Evans, J. (1971). *Living with a man who is dying.* New York: Taplinger Publishing.

Fox, S. S., & Scherl, D. J. (1972). Crisis intervention with victims of rape. *Social Work, 17,* 37–42.

Kubler-Ross, E. (1969). *On death and dying.* New York: Macmillan.

Lindemann, E. (1965). Symptomatology and management of acute grief. In H. J. Parad (Ed.) *Crisis intervention: Selected readings.* (pp. 7–21). New York: Family Service Association of America. (Reprinted from *American Journal of Psychiatry,* 1944, *101.*)

Prichard, E. R., Collard, J., Orcutt, B. A., Kutscher, A. H., Seeland, I., & Lefkowitz, N. (Eds.). (1977). *Social work with the dying patient and the family.* New York: Columbia University Press.

Shneidman, E., & Farberow, N. L. (Eds.). (1957). *Clues to suicide.* New York: McGraw-Hill.

Verwoerdt, A. (1966). Death and the family. *Medical Opinion and Review, 1* (12), 38–43.

Walker, J. I. (1983). *Psychiatric emergencies intervention and resolution.* Philadephia: J. B. Lippincott.

7

Family and Life Cycles

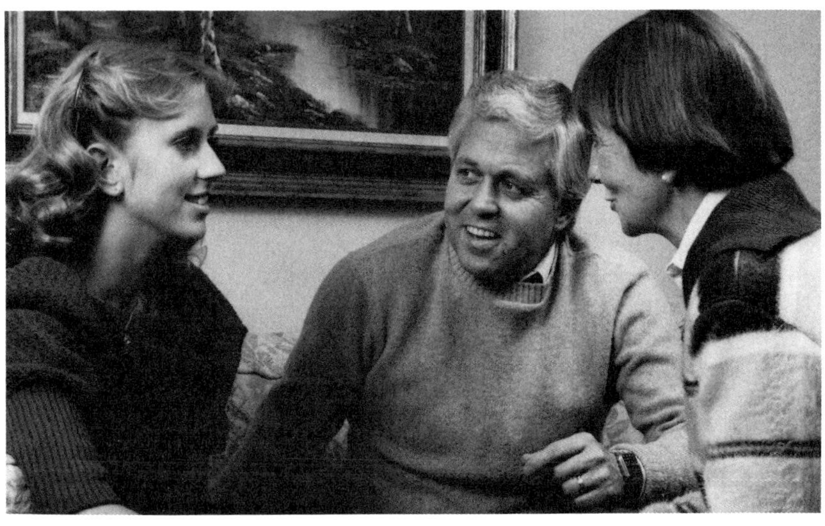

The discussion thus far has focused on the individual in crisis. This chapter will expand our knowledge and understanding of crisis theory and techniques to include the family and certain life cycle crises, specifically, adolescence, middle age, and old age. These times of the life cycle seem to be common points for the development of crises because of significant psychological and biological changes that occur at the same time.

The underlying definition of the family in crisis is the same as for the individual. That is, the family is assumed to be in equilibrium and functioning satisfactorily until a significant event occurs that threatens its stability. The event is perceived to be so dangerous to family stability and functioning that the family's usual coping methods are ineffective, causing a crisis. More will be said about this later.

A life cycle crisis is caused by an individual's inability to successfully adapt to the tasks and changes brought on by maturation (see Erikson [1963] for the adaptive tasks of each phase of the life cycle).

Again, crisis in this context means functional debilitation or ineffectiveness resulting from the occurrence of some event, in this case the events and condition of the aging process. It does not mean the characteristic upset associated with all significant changes in life, as in the popular use of the phrase "middle-age crisis."

THE FAMILY

A family is an organized system of interacting personalities with characteristic ways of functioning. It has several important functions. The first function of the family is the socialization of its children. Next comes the satisfaction of the emotional and affectional needs of its members. The family provides love and security, which we know are critical to psychic development and social functioning. Third, the family is an economic unit that ensures the physical survival of its members. Finally, the family ensures the continuity of society by incorporating the society's values, traditions, and laws into its system.

The family system is responsible for meeting these four basic purposes. Let us briefly review how a family system develops as a first step in understanding family functioning. A marriage, the prelude to a family begins when a man and a woman from different families legally agree to live together. They agree to attempt to meet each other's needs. These two people bring to this relationship their own socialization experiences, their own individual psychic systems, and their idiosyncratic needs, expectations, and ways of loving, giving, and receiving. To be successful in marriage they must fuse their individual psychic systems into one; at the same time each must maintain his and her own identity and individuality. To do this well, both partners need to agree on and adjust to new roles, a somewhat difficult task. Much of the conflict found in marriages and families is caused by people losing or being confused about their own identities. We saw an example of this in the case of Anne (see chapter 2), who felt considerable conflict over being "just" a housewife and mother and wanted to get a job so she could feel worthwhile.

If marriage requires psychological adjustments and adaptations, the birth of children requires even greater change. For one thing, there are two additional roles to fulfill: those of mother and father. However, the need for personal identity and individuality never changes. How an individual functions as a mother or father is influenced by childhood relationships with parents, by personality development, and by individual needs, feelings, and goals, all subject to change as the individual passes through the life cycle. As a unit, each family joins the diverse backgrounds and traits of its members to develop habitual patterns of functioning and coping with life stresses. Each family also develops needs, values, and goals. Like the individual, each family will develop specific behavioral patterns that it uses to achieve its goals, to meet its needs, and to adhere to its values. At the same time, the family, just as the individual, must deal with events that threaten its equilibrium (e.g., a child being unjustly picked on at school, an illness of one of its members). As long as the family can satisfactorily function, equilibrium can be maintained. To keep equilibrium, each family develops a homeostatic process. Riskin (1963) supports this view, stating:

> The family is viewed as an ongoing system. It tends to maintain itself around some point of equilibrium which has been established as the family evolves. The system is a dynamic, not a static, one. There is a continuous process of input into the system, and thus a tendency for the system to be pushed away from the equilibrium point. . . . Over a period of time, the family develops certain repetitive, enduring techniques, or patterns of interaction for maintaining its equilibrium when confronted by stress. This development tends to hold whether the stress is internal or external, acute or chronic, trivial or gross. Those techniques, which are assumed to be characteristic for a given family, are regarded as homeostatic mechanisms.

Family As a System

A family can be easily understood as a social system. Olsen (1968) defines a social system very clearly:

> A social system is a model of social organization that possesses a distinctive total unit beyond its component parts, that is distinguished from its environment by a clearly defined boundary whose subunits are at least partially interrelated within relatively stable patterns of social order. Put even more simply, a social system is a bounded set of interrelated activities that together constitute a single entity.

The concept of the family as a system implies that a change in one member brings about a corresponding change in the rest of the system; in this case, the other members. Each member has a different role and function. The quality of the functioning of any overall system depends on the functioning of the largest subsystem. In the case of the family, this is the marital pair. The marriage is the heart of the family, and all other subsystems revolve around it. It is the basis for understanding the organizational structure of the family as well as the dynamic interaction of its members. The family system also develops rules and procedures to keep it organized and to guide it in fulfilling its purpose and functions. There are dynamic forces—emotional exchanges—that govern the emotional and affectional atmosphere of the family.

To understand a family's structure and functioning, we will look at its communication and interaction patterns.

Family in Crisis

All families experience upsetting events, and all of them have some degree of strength to cope with the stress. However, some upsetting events produce a crisis in some families and not in others. Goldstein and Giddings (1973) state:

> A crisis-proof family must have agreement in its role structure, satisfaction of the physical and emotional needs of its members, and goals toward which the family is moving collectively. Having all of those, the family is adequately organized and has crisis-meeting resources. Lacking them, the family is inadequately organized and likely to prove vulnerable to crisis-precipitating events. If a family has deficiencies in crisis-meeting resources, they will tend to experience and define hazardous circumstances as crisis.

While Goldstein and Giddings place a great deal of the responsibility for a family developing crisis on its structure, we should realize that the development of any crisis, family or individual, does not depend solely on the strength of the family or individual. It depends on the subjective meaning of the event. This means that any family or person has the potential to develop a crisis if the right event occurs, regardless of strength. As stated in chapter 1, crisis theory confirms human vulnerability to stress. History is replete with examples of people overcoming the greatest of hardships only to succumb to the most common events.

A family in crisis is defined as a functionally debilitated family system. The crisis is precipitated by its reaction to some event perceived to be so dangerous to its existence or to its equilibrium that it is unable to fulfill its functions or to meet the needs of its members. Consequently, the family's reaction to the event leaves the members feeling helpless and unable to function as effectively as they did before the event. Although in a family crisis each member is affected individually and each member's method of coping varies, it is the threat to total family functioning that is the major focus. Family crises develop from two basic sources: external and internal events. External precipitating events are natural catastrophes, death, illness, the birth of a handicapped child, and so forth. External events, as a rule, do not tear the family apart emotionally as do internal events, although they can. In most cases, external events cause the family to band closer together. However, the crisis is caused by the family's perception and interpretation of the event as being dangerous to its existence as a unit, and its lacking the capacity and resources to adequately handle the situation. Internal precipitating events are those that are caused by one or more members of the family threatening the internal functioning, emotional equilibrium, or values, goals, or existence of the family as an integral unit. Examples of internal precipitating events are the mental illness of a member, changes in role relationships and status, an adolescent running away, a child leaving home, infidelity, the introduction of a new member to the family system, and so forth. The field of family therapy is based on internal precipitating events. Although we have classified precipitating events of family crises, it should be emphasized that any event can precipitate a crisis in the family if it is perceived to be dangerous to its existence or to its internal functioning.

Treatment of Family in Crisis

The concern about family instability has become a national interest, as evidenced by the rapid growth of the family therapy field. There are many different approaches to understanding and treating the family. Table 7.1 shows the numerous schools of family therapy and their historical antecedents. The frame of reference provided here is constructed to further one's understanding of treatment of people in crisis. It is not meant to go beyond crisis treatment; however, it can be supplemented with other schools of family therapy.

Crisis As a Family Problem

The first step in family crisis treatment is to establish clearly that the problem is a family problem. Regardless of the precipitating event and who appears to be responsible, it has to be understood that the precipitating event affects all of the family members. This means that all family members capable of contributing to family functioning should be included in the session. Sometimes a parent or older child will say, "It's Mike with the problem, so why do I have to come?" The answer is, of course, is that it is a *family* problem, affecting all the members and how they are getting along with each other and carrying out their responsibilities. If very young children are not contributing to or reacting to the crisis, they may be left out of subsequent sessions. Most families in crisis are eager to participate. They may have felt a great deal of self-blame and guilt long before they appear for help. Once the crisis is perceived to be a family problem, the next step for the therapist is to establish rapidly a constructive relationship with the family. This means that the therapist relates positively to each member at the same time that the members may be competing with each other for the therapist's support.

It is important for each family member to feel that the therapist is an ally. Hence the therapist must appear as a helping person to all. This requires considerable skill, especially in families with a definite political power structure. The therapist has to guard against overidentifying with one member. In some agencies for runaway adolescents, for example, therapists tend to overidentify with the adolescent to the point that the parents are often alienated. In child guidance clinics some

TABLE 7.1 *Historical antecedents of family therapy approaches: Theorists*

Humanistic	*Psychoanalytic–Psychodynamic*	*Behavioral*	*Systems*
Phenomenology	Historical,	Historical, Classical	A. Korzybsky
G. Hegel	Orthodox	E. Kraeplin	J. Dewey and M.
E. Husserl	S. Freud	P. Janet	Bentley
M. Heidegger	A. Adler	J. B. Watson	L. von Bertanlanffy
K. Jaspers	C. Jung	L. Thorndyke	G. Bateson
L. Binswanger	O. Rank	J. R. Kantor	J. Ruesch
D. Syngg and	W. Reich	Drive	D. D. Jackson
H. W. Coombs	M. Klein	C. L. Hull	J. Spiegel
C. R. Rogers	O. Fenichel	E. Miller and	
K. F. Riegel and	A. Freud	J. Dollard	
dialectics	Interpersonal–	K. W. Spence	
Existentialism	Adaptational	J. Wolpe	
S. Kierkegaard	H. Hartmann	T. A. Stampf	
J. P. Sartre	K. Horney	H. J. Eysenck	
A. H. Maslow	E. Fromm	Reinforcement	
V. E. Frankl	A. Meyer	B. F. Skinner	
R. D. Laing	H. S. Sullivan	S. W. Bijou	
R. May	S. Rado	T. Ayllon	
S. Jourard	Modern–Day	N. H. Azrin	
Experientialism	Revisionists	Social Learning	
J. Moreno and	E. H. Erikson and	A. Bandura	
psychodrama	stages of	J. B. Rotter	
F. Perls and	development	F. Kanfer	
gestalt school	R. R. Grinker, Sr.	L. P. Ullman	
G. Murphy and	and		
W. C. Schutz	transactional		
G. Bach and fight	viewpoint		
training	E. Berne and		
I. Rolf and holistic	transactional		
movement	analysis		
expressivists,	A. Fairburn and		
body:	British object		
A. Lowen	relations		
Detachers-	school		
meditators:			
A. Watts			
Communicators:			
R. Bandler			
and J.			
Grinder			

Note. From *Approaches to Family Therapy* by James C. Hansen and Lucianne L'Abate, 1982. Macmillan Publishing Co., Inc., New York, Collier Macmillan Publishers, London. Reprinted by permission.

parents' self-blame keeps them from perceiving the part their children play in the family problem.

Focus on Precipitating Event and Identify Problem for Family. While the family is gathering, the therapist watches their seating arrangements, looking for possible significant patterns. Once the family is gathered, the task of the therapist is to elicit and encourage the expression of whatever affect or emotion is present. If none is present at the time, the therapist can begin by discussing the precipitating event. If discussing the precipitating event brings out feelings, each member should be encouraged to ventilate them before pursuing the precipitating event further. The therapist should pay particular attention to who speaks first and how that is determined. The therapist should observe the members' different perspectives, especially if there are differences between mother and father or parent and child. In addition, the therapist should get everyone's views and reactions.

Generally, the family will respond differently to external precipitating events than to internal ones. As previously stated, they tend to band together in the face of external events and are probably easier to work with as a total unit. In such cases the therapist must understand how the event is perceived by each family member. Consequently, the therapist should get everyone's view and reaction. Individual family members may react to the reaction of other family members, not specifically to the event itself. This is especially true of children. If the family crisis is precipitated by the loss of a loved one and all family members are not grieving appropriately, the therapist should encourage those who are not to express painful feelings. It should be remembered that family crises precipitated by external events pose a threat to family existence as a unit as well as the threat to love relationships and affectional tendencies. Consequently, eliciting and encouraging the expression of painful feelings and the meaning of the event to each family member is a major therapeutic task.

Internal precipitating events caused by a family member that threaten family equilibrium and functioning are more complex and require the therapist to intervene in the family's patterns of interaction. Consider the following example:

Mr. and Mrs. Sargent brought their 16-year-old son John to the crisis center for help before they put him out of the home. The problem was precipitated by John physically attacking his mother for not letting him have the car. Mr. Sargent stated that John's attacking his mother was a sign that he was dangerous and had a "screw loose." John and his mother have not gotten along for the past three years. Since John received his driver's license, the relationship between him and his mother has grown destructively worse. However, this was the first time that he had physically attacked her.

In a case like this, what is the real precipitating event? We know that on the surface it was John not being able to get the car. Did John's mother provoke him beyond his capacity to not react? What was there about this situation that was so threatening to the family system that the parents wanted to handle it by removing John if he could not continue to function as expected in spite of his movement toward independence? As we can see, a family crisis can be precipitated when habitual patterns of functioning are threatened. Although a family is an organized system, within its structure it must have room for change. John's movement toward independence was a threat to the family equilibrium. His parents were not ready for change. A family must be ready for change in the dynamic interrelationships and roles of its members brought on by life cycles. The precipitating event provides significant clues to the nature of family functioning.

Determine Nuclear Problem. The next step in working with the family crisis is to determine the nuclear problem. In the case of the Sargent family we know that something happened that was extremely significant to John, since this was the first time he had ever attacked his mother. A discussion of feelings and events leading up to the precipitating event can help to illuminate the nuclear problem. Was his mother trying to maintain her control over John? Was she angry at her husband? What is the nature of their relationship? Is John being used to hide a poor marital relationship threatened by his impending emancipation? These questions and others are answered as the family members talk and communicate with each other. As the session progresses, the focus of the family moves from the precipitating event to intrafamilial feelings, behavior, and interactions.

It is by looking at the family communication process and interactions that the family is understood and the nuclear problem is manifested. As the therapist observes and listens he or she discovers the nuclear problem; that is, the underlying cause of the family's crisis.

Assess and Evaluate Family Structure and Functioning. As when working with the individual in crisis, assessment and evaluation of the family begins with the first contact. By now the therapist has a wealth of information on which to base assessment and evaluation. This phase properly begins with identifying family structure. This is important for evaluating the family's potential for fulfilling its purpose and functions. Generally, family structure consists of a mother, father, and one or more children. A crisis can be precipitated by a threat to family structure such as the introduction of a new member or the loss of a member. The single-parent family is vulnerable to the development of a crisis because of a deficit in structure. It is deprived of a resource that generally gives strength and support to family structure. The strength of family structure is determined by how each member fulfills functions and roles. In this regard the heart of family functioning is the marriage. The therapist assesses the contribution of the marital relationship to the family crisis. What is the relationship between husband and wife? Are they together or disunited and competitive? A divided family cannot be a strong family. Is the marriage an unwillfully dominate and submissive relationship? Revolving around the marital relationship are the functions and roles of the children. What are the children's roles and expectations individually and collectively? Are they perceived as respected individuals, or are they used by one or both parents? If so, how and in what way? For example, is one a scapegoat who is keeping the family from total disintegration? What is the nature of feelings and emotional atmosphere in the family? What is the nature of the communication process? How does each member feel about the others and about the relationship of others in the family? What needs are being met in the family? What needs are not being met, and how are members reacting to unmet needs? In sum, the assessment and evaluation of the family requires the evaluation of the family as a total unit and of each individual's contribution to its total functioning. The therapist needs to answer such questions in order to know the degree of debilitation and what areas of family functioning have been affected. Furthermore, it identifies areas of weakness requiring treatment and sources of strength than can be used to help reestablish equilibrium and strengthen family functioning. Synthesizing this information enables the therapist to formulate a dynamic explanation of the causes of the family crisis.

Provide Family with Self-Understanding. By this time, some of the upset should be reduced, and the therapist can move to cognitive restoration. In this phase the crisis therapist will give the family an explanation of the cause and reasons for the family crisis. The therapist should identify the positive and negative aspects of the family functioning, as revealed in how they communicate. He also can identify various role assignments, their consequences, and why they are no longer functional, thereby causing family conflict. Hence the therapist helps the family move toward new roles.

Plan and Implement Treatment. If the precipitating event involves a threat to overall functioning, the family must be helped to work through threats of its disintegration. For example, if the crisis is caused by the loss of a member on whom the family depended for survival, they must be helped to grieve as a group and individually. In all aspects of therapy with a family in crisis, the therapist must access and use the strengths of the family. The therapist should identify a potential leader as a source of strength for reequalizing or reintegrating the family as a whole system. Every group, to be functional, must have a leader.

In the subsequent treatment sessions, the family as a group must agree to work together to continue to resolve the crisis; that is, to change roles, rules, and so forth, that will facilitate growth and restrengthening. If the precipitating event is a loss of a family member, then the task is to complete the grieving process and directly or indirectly delegate another family member to assume the unfilled roles and responsibilities. If the family crisis is a life cycle problem, such as a child leaving home or resistance to the emancipation of children, the family must be helped to cope with such a disequalizing event and to reintegrate in another acceptable fashion. By this time each member should be aware of his or her own significance and responsibility to the family. Family members then should be willing to compromise for the sake of the group.

Termination and Follow-Up. The family is ready for termination of therapy when the crisis is resolved and the family has returned to a precrisis level of functioning. It is to be hoped that they have learned a great deal about themselves as a family and individually and that they have also learned new ways to resolve problems. At the point of termination, the family should be advised that they will be contacted in a specific period of time (one month, three months, six months) to learn how they are doing. This not only suggests an interest, but it also suggests that help is available if another crisis occurs. If the crisis is resolved but long-term therapy is indicated, referral should be made. The success of such a suggestion depends on how it is presented. After one to six sessions (or one to six weeks) with a family, the therapist has a great deal of knowledge about them. The way a referral is recommended should be based on this knowledge of why the referral is necessary and what it may accomplish.

CRISIS PRECIPITATED BY MARITAL SEPARATION AND DIVORCE

The most stressful life events are the death of a spouse, divorce, and martial separation (Holmes and Rahe, 1967). Both separation and divorce are increasing at an alarming rate, and many of these events will become crises requiring intervention. Intervention at the point of crisis can prevent long-term negative effects and make adjustment smoother.

Many explanations exist for marital choice, but the principal reason is a function of personality development influenced by experiences with one's parents and their marriage. When two people agree to marry, their egos fuse and each becomes an internal part of the other's psychic system. Consequently, when a unilateral decision to separate or divorce takes place, the non-consenting mate generally reacts to the loss with depression, grief and mourning because it is as if that mate has lost a part of himself or herself (Counts and Sacks, 1985). Whether the reactions to separation and divorce become a crisis depends on a number of factors:

a. The intrapsychic meaning of the lost spouse to the non-consenting mate. A crisis is likely to occur if the latter relies abnormally upon the former for psychic equilibrium, identity, and self-esteem.
b. Whether the non-consenting mate experienced significant losses in early childhood.
c. The nature of the circumstances leading to the separation and divorce; the significance of the circumstances will be determined by the non-consenting spouse's own interpretations of the meaning, which can result in guilt feelings, self-blame, and self-denigration.
d. Economic dependency on the part of the non-consenting spouse.

In cases where economic dependency is the precipitating event, the therapist should address the economic problems, but other reasons should also be explored.

Assessment and Evaluation

The non-consenting spouse is the person in crisis and the one who usually first comes to the therapist alone. The meaning of the precipitating event is generally the pain of loss or threatened loss of a significant loved one and all other essentials associated with marriage and the family. After discussing the precipitating event, the therapist should gather information that will help the therapist to understand the client better. It is important that we understand the personal history of the spouse in crisis since marriage is a function of personality development. Past relationships and life "scripts" may be a part of the problem. The crisis reaction may be the result of past experiences with significant loved ones—especially losses of loved ones. Consequently, the more historical information we can gather, the better we can understand the spouse in crisis and the meaning and contributing factors of the precipitating event. A history of the courtship and marriage are particularly important in understanding needs, motivation, and maturity level. The client may have experienced romantic fantasies which have become nightmarish realities. By exploring these early phases of the relationship, the therapist can learn about the client's reasons for marrying, what needs he or she expected to have met at that time, and how these needs changed over time. Take the case of Becky and Matt. Matt wanted a divorce because Becky was no longer the same woman he had married. When he married her, she was an 18-year-old high school graduate and he was a 21-year-old college senior. At that time, she admired his intellectual ability and thought he was the most intelligent person in the world. He would talk to her for hours while she listened, captivated by his every word. After a few years of marriage Becky returned to college, an experience that changed the way she perceived and related to Matt. She discovered that the world was filled with ideas other than his, some of which were ideas of her own, and which at time conflicted with Matt's. As a result of her growth, they often argued and disagreed. One day Matt informed Becky that he wanted a divorce. Becky's reaction was a crisis condition: although she had altered her perceptual, economic, and intellectual dependence on Matt, she had not changed her emotional dependence and psychological need for him.

As we can see from the case of Becky and Matt, needs change. If a marriage is motivated by either transitory needs, an attempt to resolve intrapsychic conflicts through negative complementaries, or to escape an intolerable environment, the passage of time carries with it the chance that spouses will change, one of the two coming to feel that the other cannot meet his or her needs.

Treatment

After the initial interview with the spouse in crisis, the therapist can recommend a treatment plan. Such a plan should begin with the therapist seeing the couple together; if a family is involved, the therapist should see together all members old enough to contribute to family functioning. Everyone should be encouraged to discuss openly the precipitating event and the feelings associated with it, thus facilitating the grief process as much as possible. The goal is to help each family member accept the inevitable while experiencing the grieving process and tending to the necessities as effectively as possible. The therapist should make every effort to prevent any family member from exhibiting destructive or acting-out behavior. Treatment for the crisis of separation and divorce should help the client work through associated feelings, accept the reality of the necessary changes in living brought about by the event, and begin planning for life to continue. During the treatment stage, the therapist must keep in mind and prepare for the fact that stress produced by separation and divorce usually lasts longer than the crisis. At the conclusion of crisis treatment, the therapist should assess whether any family member is experiencing psychological conflicts that prevent adjustment to the distress of this event. That member should be referred to traditional psychotherapy and all family members should be made aware of additional services that they may use at any time in the future.

THE LIFE CYCLE

The life cycle is the maturational sequence each person goes through during the normal passage from birth to death. Each phase involves certain psychological tasks and adaptations to certain biological conditions. Phases are not discrete; there is some overlapping. The success achieved in each phase is related to the success attained in each previous phase. Common phases of the life cycle are shown in Figure 7.1.

Erikson (1959) refers to each phase of the life cycle as a crisis:

> Each state becomes a crisis because incipient growth and awareness in a significant part function goes together with a shift in instinctual energy and yet causes specific vulnerability in that part. One of the most difficult questions to decide, therefore, is whether or not a child at a given stage is weak or strong. Perhaps it would be best to say that he is always vulnerable in some respects and completely oblivious and insensitive in others, but that at the same time he is unbelievably persistent in the same respect in which he is vulnerable.

Erikson uses the term *crisis* as a problem-solving process. The term is appropriate because of the vulnerability of people at various phases of the life cycle, particularly those that are turning points. Although a crisis can develop at any point in the cycle, we will discuss three vulnerable phases: adolescence, middle adulthood, and late adulthood.

According to the life cycle model, all that is needed to understand human behavior is to compare the behavior of the individual with the expected behavior of the appropriate phase of the person's life cycle according to chronological age. But chronological age is less important in understanding behavior than is the individual's emotional maturity. Chronological age provides only a baseline; it lets you know the adaptative task the person should be working on. In other words, a person's

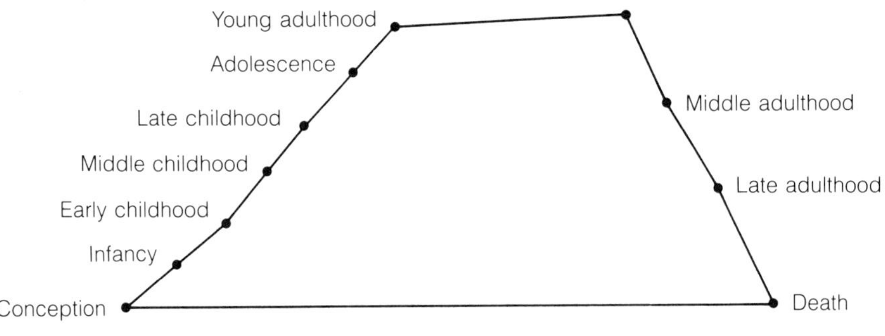

Figure 7.1 Life Cycle

specific behavior and feelings indicate where he or she is *emotionally*, according to the life cycle model. If a middle-aged man feels and acts like an adolescent is expected to feel and act, adolescence is his emotional level. Of course, in mature psychic functioning the individual's feelings and behavior are reasonably consistent with position in the life cycle.

Adolescence

An adolescent in crisis creates a family crisis. At times, the adolescent engages in crisis-producing behavior as a means of trying to restore family equilibrium. Consider the following example:

Sixteen-year-old Jack called the crisis center requesting an appointment. When he was seen he said that he was distressed by the way that he was getting along with his mother. The conflict between the two was getting unbearable. She was always criticizing the work he did at home and school. He had no freedom to do the things that the rest of his friends did. For instance, he could not use the family car. She picked at him all of the time, and their relationship had begun to affect her marriage, since his father defended Jack when he was at home. The crisis therapist saw this as a family problem. She and Jack agreed that the whole family should be called in; however, the mother refused. Some two weeks later, Jack ran away. He was gone for a little over a month. As he kept on the move, he would call his dad or write a postcard letting him know that he was all right. After weeks of roaming around the nation, he went to his uncle's home in Florida. When his parents picked him up, they agreed to seek family treatment.

We will discuss some of the common problems of adolescence that cause crises for adolescents themselves. But before discussing the adolescent in crisis, let's review some characteristics of adolescent development to help distinguish between average expectable adolescent turbulence and the adolescent in crisis.

Adolescence is the individual's total psychosocial reaction and adaptation to puberty. Puberty is the biological event of sexual maturation, during which full genital and reproductive maturity are reached. Adolescence generally begins around the age of 13 years and continues until full independence is achieved. Thus the conclusion of adolescence can vary considerably; it is not solely the function of chronological age. For example, the person who goes to work right after high school may be independent and assume adult responsibilities four years before someone who goes to college and remains dependent on his or her parents.

In general, the assumption of adult responsibilities marks the conclusion of adolescence as long as sexual maturation is complete. Three factors influence adolescent development in Western society: (a) biological and physical changes, (b) resultant changes in the psychic system, and (c) the social environment, specifically parents and the culture. We will briefly consider all three.

Adolescents and Biological Changes The onset of adolescence is marked by puberty, which in turn is manifested by the first appearance of secondary sex characteristics and marked physical changes and growth. Puberty in girls (which occurs earlier than in boys) involves the appearance of pubic hair, the enlargement of breasts and nipples, the growth of genitalia, and most significantly, menarche (the first menstrual period). Most American girls reach puberty between the ages of 10 and 16 years. Engel (1962) states:

> On the average, there is a lapse of two to four years after menarche before ovulation finally takes place and conception becomes possible. Full reproductive capacity in the girl is not achieved for another two to four years after ovulation has been initiated.

Engel's statement refers to a statistical average; girls as young as 11 years have borne children.

The onset of puberty in boys is marked by a rapid growth spurt, muscular development, voice change, genital growth, and appearance of pubic and facial hair. It occurs around the ages of 12 to 14 years, some two years later than in girls. However, boys' changes are very rapid, and their physical strength and growth in height generally occur very rapidly also.

Throughout adolescence, girls move toward emotional adulthood more quickly than boys do. They are generally attracted to older boys rather than boys of the same age. Each adolescent's pattern of internal growth is inconsistent; this often gives them the feeling of strangeness or awkwardness. As Blos (1962) states:

> This lack of uniformity in physical development, called *asymmetrical growth*, often puts extreme demands upon the physical and mental adaptivity of the individual.

This asymmetrical growth not only makes it difficult for many adolescents to control their bodies, but it affects body image as well and influences the degree to which adolescents compete and make comparisons with their peers.

This is only a brief description of the human biological and physical changes that occur at the onset of puberty. These changes greatly affect the adolescent's psychic functioning, often making average expectable behavior turbulent. However, it is not solely physical changes and sexual maturation that make adolescence so difficult. The difficulty is also caused by changes in the psychic system.

Adolescent Psychic System. By the time the child reaches adolescence, most of his or her growth and development have taken place. The child has had a wealth of experiences, all contributing bits and pieces to the psychic system. During the relative quiet periods of middle and late childhood, the psychic system has been integrating and solidifying an enormous amount of learning and achievement. The child has had a great many experiences in dealing with the social environment, especially in relating to peers and the school and other institutions, and generally with the support of parents. As stated earlier, human development is an evolutionary process in which the success of each phase depends on success in the preceding phases. Consequently, the individual's ability to cope with adolescence basically depends on the degree of success during preceding phases of growth and maturation. But regardless of the quality of psychosocial development before adolescence, some conflict and problems are inevitable. The onset of adolescence in many ways dismantles and rearranges some of the parts of a psychic system that has been completed over a number of years. This system served the child well while the child was growing up in a variable social environment. Now the system must withstand the onslaught of the turbulence and confusion of adolescence However, this final renovation of the psychic system before adulthood offers the individual the opportunity to enter adulthood stronger and more capable. It also provides the opportunity to turn back if the individual is not quite ready, although the time it takes to make the decision will vary from child to child.

The psychic system at adolescence is a mixture of strength, weakness, and potential. The adolescent's ego is stronger than the child's because of experiences and cognitive development. A wealth of ego capacities have now completely matured (i.e., cognition, memory, perception, mobility, and so forth). Special talents and abilities may show up. All this creates many new ways for the adolescent to cope with stress. But at the same time the ego is stronger, adolescent needs and drives are also intensified. The adolescent sex drive and capacity have matured, giving an additional force to manage. It is important that they be handled constructively. Pubescence makes adolescents biologically equal to their parents. This can have a far-reaching effect, depending on the relationship with the parents and the make-up of the psychic system. It is a basic struggle because the sex drive and affectual needs are so strong; if the ego is not capable of handling them constructively, negative consequences can result, as we see in the increase in pregnancies among teenagers. In such cases the significance is not so much that the child had intercourse but that she got pregnant in this day of birth control pills and sex education in schools.

Another difficulty inherent in adolescence is the need for independence. This independence is facilitated by the partial turning away from parents. Some of the ego strength already gained is reduced as the adolescent turns away from the reliable support of parents. After having internalized into his or her psychic system the parents' love, experiences, values, and ways of perceiving and thinking, the only way the adolescent feels adultlike and independent is by behaving and feeling, to varying degrees, in ways quite opposite from those of parents. The length of time the child has spent depending on the parents and their closeness contribute to this end. As the adolescent turns away from parents, a very valuable source of support is lost and the adolescent attempts to replace them with new people at the same time. This contributes to adolescents' not knowing who they are. It may lead to adolescents turning inward and becoming quite self-centered. At the same time that this change in ego support is going on, a change in the functioning of conscience is also going on. Recall that the conscience was internalized from the experiences with parents. The child learned right and wrong, good and bad, and moral values from them. When adolescents turn away from parents, they also turn away from conscience. The conscience has also been an internal measure of parental approval and a component of self-esteem. Adolescents experience this turning away in a way similar to mourning; they may feel that they have lost a loved one. This accounts for their frequent feelings of depression, moodiness, and loneliness. The degree and extent of this depression depend on the degree of hostility previously developed toward the parents (Brenner, 1973). In understanding this, keep in mind that early relationships with parents form the basis of the development of the ego and conscience. During adolescence, memories of these early relationships are reactivated and the adolescent begins to react to them or defend against them. The greater the early hostility, the more difficult it is for the adolescent to deal with the original feelings that are now reactivated. Consequently the turning away from the parents is confused with aggression turned toward the self. The result of the hostility toward the self is depression. Whether it is a customary depression or a neurotic or psychotic depression, an adolescent's acting out or antisocial behavior combines the hostility originally directed toward the parents with other forms of disturbances.

The conscience functioning learned from parents is now temporarily abandoned. As a consequence, not only does the adolescent feel a loss of love, but he or she also feels a reduction in sources of control, evaluation, and prevention. This lets the adolescent engage in unusual or uncharacteristic behavior that ordinarily conscience would prevent. It is common for most adolescents to engage in some semidelinquent or rebellious behavior or behavior that is generally out of character or unexpected. However, in Western society it seems that each adolescent must go through this to some degree in order to become relatively independent of parents, to begin to establish identity and become a responsible adult.

The whole adolescent process leads to adulthood and independent functioning. The helplessness of human beings, the lengthy time of dependency, and the resultant affectional bond all make the movement from childhood to adulthood a painful one in spite of the happiness associated with it. The child must work this out in his or her own way, and the decision to move toward adulthood causes ambivalence. Although the adolescent wants to be an adult, he or she also wants to be able to remain a child.

A wide range of adolescent behavior is considered to be average expectable (normal). There is danger, however, when an adolescent's ego is too weak to adequately handle emerging drives, specifically the sex drive. The adolescent can handle this in two harmful ways: (a) early marriage at the expense of prematurely resolidfying the psychic system, or (b) excessive use of repression (Blos, 1962). In getting married prematurely, the adolescent is deprived of certain dependency gratification and is thrust too quickly into adult responsibilities. The overly repressed adolescent is emotionally shallow, making it difficult for him or her to develop genuine interpersonal relationships and to be able to enjoy pleasures of life.

Even though adolescence is a turbulent phase, most adolescents enter adulthood with a reasonable chance of success. Specifically, the adolescent must emotionally emancipate himself or herself from family so that an identity can be established. This means the adolescent still loves the parents and needs their love but not in the dependent way characteristic of earlier childhood. It means also that the adolescent takes the wealth of socializing experiences and synthesizes them into a form that represents self and allows the adolescent to say "I am" rather than "Who am I?" The adolescent must begin to establish a personal identity and reintegrate an adequate functioning psychic system. The adolescent must also prepare for a vocation. In addition, most adolescents must prepare for mature heterosexual relationships and for living and associating intimately with a person of the opposite sex.

Adolescence is an age of anxiety for parents as well as for the adolescent. To see a previously dependent child who was malleable and manageable become seemingly independent and rebellious is often painful for the parents. The child's lack of communication and turning away from the family can be quite an awakening for the parents. This awakening occurs on two levels. First, the parents begin to realize that they are growing older and that their child is becoming a young adult. This provokes their feelings about middle age and the speed with which their lives are passing. The greatest anxiety for parents, however, is facing their own unresolved adolescent feelings and conflicts, which are reactivated by their adolescent child. During their own adolescent years they may have been able to set aside their adolescent conflicts and struggles and achieve a certain amount of stability. However, the onset of their child's adolescent development, with all of its struggles and conflicts, reactivates the parents' old conflicts and their own struggles. The parents again need to repress their unresolved conflicts, which is generally manifested in rigid rules and regulations and renewed effort at maintaining control of the adolescent. It is also not unusual for parents to look on their adolescent child as their last chance for achievement and therefore push the child farther than the child can or wants to go. The reactivation of the parents' adolescent struggles and conflicts can show up in many forms. The important fact is that it influences how the parents relate and react to the adolescent, which in turn creates considerable family upset.

Adolescent and Society. The third important factor influencing the adolescent is society. In our society, adolescence has been a phase held in abeyance. Unlike other societies, we have no initiation rites or rites of passage, although the driver's license and limited liquor privileges are efforts in that direction. Actually, society itself contributes heavily to adolescent conflict and struggles. For example, the process of sexual maturation is a universal phenomenon; however, the psychological reactions accompanying the physiological changes are influenced by societal expectations. The pressures of this period of transition create strong emotions that the adolescent must cope with in ways that conform to social conditions and expectations, or problems ensue. Although society does not help the adolescent through conflicts and struggles, he or she is still expected to emerge as a healthy and happy adult. The easiest way to cope with such demands and inconsistencies is to do the opposite of what is expected: if sexual inhibition is the problem, then sexual freedom is the solution. However, since sexual freedom is the opposite of sexual inhibition, it really is not a solution, but the same coin turned over. At this point, sex education in the school is not the answer because it deals with intellectual knowledge rather than emotional reactions.

The lengthy educational process fosters dependency and a patriarchal tradition. The inconsistencies and injustices in our society are also conducive to the adolescent's turning away from society and toward idealism. But real societies do not change easily, and the adolescent must learn to react constructively to the things seen as wrong. To improve conditions, the adolescent must learn to adapt and at the same time to change what can be changed.

Adolescent in Crisis.

It is generally agreed that adolescence is a time of turbulence. However, we wish to distinguish between adolescence as an expectable phase of upset in which equilibrium is restored (even though with considerable difficulty), and a crisis as defined in this book. We are discussing an adolescent crisis as a problem that is so debilitating that outside intervention is warranted. As a rule, an adolescent crisis is a family crisis, and generally the therapist should involve the adolescent's family for the best resolution. The exception, of course, could be some of the usual upset that the adolescent experiences at school, for which the adolescent goes to the school counselor for help. At the same time, some problems for which adolescents consult school counselors are real crises and should involve the family.

There are three types of adolescent crisis: (a) inability to cope with some developmental task, reflecting intrapsychic conflict or the consequence of adolescence (i.e., sexual problems, peer relationships, academic failure); (b) inability to adjust to the rules, expectations, and demands of a social institution (i.e., school or the law); and (c) crisis precipitated by family relationships in which the adolescent attempts to handle the problem by behavior that threatens the functioning of the family, such as breaking a family rule or value by dating an unacceptable person, running away, or attempting suicide. Consider the following examples:

Alan, age 15, came to the crisis center on his own because he needed to talk with someone about a problem he was having. It was so personal that he did not want to talk to his parents about it. He had very few friends and no one else he could trust. He said that he was worried about the fact that he had an uncontrollable urge to masturbate and could not stop. He was so worried about it that he could no longer function. He felt depressed and felt that if his mother knew, she would be disappointed in him.

This was a rather benign problem, and Alan responded very well to psychological support, especially reassurance. Cognitive restoration involved relating his urge to masturbate with the degree of his feelings of loneliness. He responded very well and after five sessions had resolved his crisis and began to make friends. (When adolescents have conflict over masturbation, it is most often the fantasies during the act that cause the conflict rather than the act itself [Blos, 1962]).

David, age 15, was brought to the crisis center by his mother because he had been expelled from school for fighting. Although David's mother had called the child guidance clinic, he could not be seen there for five to six weeks. David's mother wanted to get him back into school immediately, but the school officials had said they would not let David back in school until he had sought professional help. On this basis David's mother thought the situation to be an emergency. David had a history of fighting, and until now his academic performance had been a little above average. During the session David expressed the feeling that his fighting was caused by his peers picking on him and harrassing him. He was especially sorry that he had to miss shop because that was the one class in which he was successful.

In cases like David's (the acting-out adolescent), both the individual and the environment have to be assessed and evaluated quickly. A child who generally has to act out has two basic problems: (a) poor impulse control and judgment, and (b) a feeling of being helpless or powerless to significantly influence or control the environment. Successful treatment in such cases requires intervention in both situations.

Beverly, 17, was brought to the emergency services of the mental health clinic after she made a suicide attempt by swallowing some aspirins. The act was precipitated by her parents' refusal to let her see her boyfriend, who was eight years older than she. This relationship had been a source of conflict and trouble for several months. On this particular occasion Beverly was caught after she had sneaked out to see him. Her father slapped her several times, and both parents joined together in forbidding her to ever see him again.

What made this a crisis for Beverly? The answer is that it was a family crisis precipitated by Beverly's desperate effort to solve it in the most expedient way she could think of at the time. What really made it a crisis was that Beverly's behavior threatened the internal functioning of the family. A family with teenagers must be able to adapt to the impending change in family equilibrium. Furthermore, they must be able to tolerate the "empty nest." They must be able to adapt to the change in their own sexuality, which they are made aware of by their teenager's budding sexuality. The questions in Beverly's case are whether her behavior and involvement with this older man represented a serious deficit in her psychic functioning and whether she was trying to resolve some intraphysic conflicts through this relationship. Adolescence is a time in which the person is still largely a child at the same time that he or she strives toward adulthood and independence. Sometimes adolescents need help in controlling their strong drives in order to constructively accomplish all of the developmental tasks. The family must be the source of help and support. However, if they are too threatened by the adolescent's behavior, they cannot help but make matters worse. At the same time, the adolescent crisis is very often a reflection of a deficit in family functioning or the result of a basic family problem. In cases like Beverly's. family therapy is indicated. After the crisis is resolved, referral for traditional treatment may be necessary.

Treatment of the Adolescent in Crisis. Permission from a parent is generally required to treat adolescents. Adolescents who come for treatment hoping their parents will not know about it should be informed of this requirement. Most often the treatment of an adolescent in crisis should be family crisis treatment, or it should involve both treatment of the adolescent individually and treatment of the family. In treatment of an adolescent individually and in the family, the same procedures are used as discussed in chapter 5. Treating the adolescent, however, requires a slightly different perspective. Consideration should be given to the fact that the adolescent is struggling with a conflict between dependency and independency. This means that the therapist must remain neutral; that is, not overidentify with the adults or with the adolescent. Naturally, the therapist should feel very empathic toward the client, but a natural constructive relationship and an understanding of the client's psychic system and functioning should be the therapist's goals. No doubt the adolescent will initially assume that the therapist is on the side of adults, since the therapist is an adult. However, the therapist cannot deny who he is and should not let the adolescent seduce him into anything other than understanding, accepting, and a desire to help. Being genuinely honest and natural is the best way to establish a constructive relationship with an adolescent.

After the beginning of a constructive relationship is in process, the therapist's intervention should be guided by several goals. The first is to think in terms of reinforcing the adolescent's ego functioning so he or she can more constructively handle both internal and external problems and conflicts. This can initially be done through supportive techniques and causal connecting statements. If it appears the adolescent has not learned and grown from this experience, referral for traditional therapy is indicated. In Beverly's case, did she learn from her crisis experience a way other than suicide to resolve problems? Did she learn about herself so that she can evaluate reality better?

Second, the therapist actively facilitates reality testing. This means that he or she has to help the adolescent appropriately distinguish subjective reality from objective reality, often by pointing out the difference. Adolescents are generally quite receptive to inconsistencies in their own thinking if it is considered in a supporting and understanding relationship.

Third, the therapist should work toward becoming a respected source of support, an alternate ego and conscience for the adolescent. This is done by gaining the adolescent's respect through support, fairness, and neutrality. Finally, the therapist must help the adolescent become responsible for behavior by cognitive restoration. In so doing, the therapist's interpretation of the psychological meaning of the behavior should come after a constructive relationship has been reasonably well established in the context of the crisis. Extra caution should be used when an adolescent's self-esteem has been seriously damaged. Because the line between average expectable adolescent upset and adolescent pathology is often blurred, careful evaluation of the psychic system should be done.

Adolescent Suicidal Behavior

The rate of suicide among adolescents has trippled in the past 20 years, and suicide has become the third leading cause of adolescent deaths (Marks, 1979). The increased incidence of suicide has made the public aware of the seriousness of this tragedy. The mass media have even portrayed the subtle signs of suicide and the impact on the family. Today, signals of suicidal behavior are more likely to be taken seriously, sending parents to a crisis treatment center. It follows, therefore, that adolescent suicidal behavior is a crisis reaction to family dysfunctioning.

Causes of Adolescent Suicidal Behavior

Adolescence is characterized by crisis, but not all adolescents react with suicidal behavior. The question is: what causes some adolescents and not others to resort to suicidal behavior as a reaction to the occurrence of upsetting events? (e.g., you can't have the family car tonight). It appears that a number of factors contribute to adolescent suicidal behavior. We will discuss three: development, family dysfunctioning, and social factors.

Adolescent Development. The major developmental problems for suicidal adolescents are the crisis of identity and identity diffusion (Erikson, 1980). The suicidal adolescent experiences greater confusion over identity at the beginning of adolescence because he or she is developmentally arrested at an earlier emotional level. As Sands and Dixon (1986) state: "It is difficult to come to terms with one's identity when one remains psychologically bound to one's parents, does not trust others, or feels inferior to others. For these adolescents, identity cannot be well established unless they deal with problems originating in the past."

Because suicidal adolescents are psychologically immature, they are not able to struggle with the process of identity development in ways that are positive to them or their parents. (The nature of this condition will be made clear in the section on family functioning.) Contributing to suicidal adolescent developmental immaturities is the problem of separation-individuation (Mahler, Pine, Bergman, 1975). Separation-individuation is the gradual process by which the child separates from the parents without totally repudiating them or himself or herself but in such a way that the child feels emotionally independent of them. This process starts early in life and is basically completed near the end of adolescence; it is marked by the ability of the adolescent to take more and more positive responsibility and gradually to reduce dependence on parents when and where appropriate. Because of the nature of family structures and functioning, separation-individuation is difficult for the suicidal adolescent. Although it may sound paradoxical, separation for the suicidal adolescent is extremely threatening—not only because it is resisted by parents, a reaction creating feelings of guilt and inadequacy, but because it gives the adolescent a feeling of extreme loneliness, of not having human connection. The developmental problem of suicidal adolescents makes them vulnerable to separation and loss, which they experience as rejection. For these individuals, the continued dependency on parents affects self-esteem, worth, and value because of the nature of the family dysfunctioning. They interpret the expectations, demands, and criticism by the parents as rejection because they feel they cannot meet the standards and thus attempt to function in their own adolescent world. In addition, this adolescent feels angry because he or she has failed to meet the seemingly impossible demands of the parents; in turn, the adolescent either internalizes the anger and becomes depressed, or acts out.

As the adolescent's effort to cope with the increasing individual and family problems fails, suicidal behavior is the only way to escape the unbearable feelings of being rejected, unloved, and worthless.

The Family System of Suicidal Adolescents. Underlying and long-standing family problems have kept the suicidal adolescent from appropriate emotional maturation. Family disintegration and unhealthy psychological functioning contribute to adolescent suicidal behavior (Cosand, Bourque, and Krave, 1982; Tishler, MacKenry, and Morgan, 1981). All through life, the suicidal adolescent has tried to meet needs in a dysfunctional family system. At the same time, the suicidal adolescent, out of need for love and dependency, maintains a strong attachment to the dysfunctional family in which communication patterns, rules, and interactions are conflicting and confusing (Sands and Dixon, 1986).

Several characteristics of the suicidal adolescent's family are consistently observed: The first is a closed system (Richman, 1971). Such family functioning prevents outside influence which threatens family equilibrium and boundaries. In particular, friends of the adolescent are a constant source of conflict because they challenge family values; they are perceived as bad, as living an undesirable lifestyle. The parents are unaware that the rejection of the adolescent's friends is a rejection of the adolescent because the choice of friends is made according to feelings of acceptance and perception of self-concept. The second characteristic of the suicidal adolescent's family is marital conflict. The marriage is the heart of family functioning. In suicidal families, marital interaction is one of anger and conflict (Pfeffer, 1981). Arguments, disagreements, and threats of separation are constant; the pervasive atmosphere is one of depression and gloom. The suicidal adolescent, being the scapegoat, believes that he or she is the cause of family problems. In reality, it only seems that way because so much turmoil is caused by the adolescent's unacceptable behavior; however, this form of adolescent behavior is a way of diverting attention from the problems in the marriage (Richman, 1971). The adolescent feels responsible for keeping the family together, but at the same time he or she is experiencing pain so intolerable that the adolescent eventually reaches a point where suicide seems to be the only escape. A third characteristic is the parents' persistent, inordinate ties to their own families and unresolved childhood problems (Pfeffer, 1981). The parents' own problems form "negative fit" which sustains the conflicts and problems. As Sands and Dixon (1986) state,

> A consequence of residues of the parents' own childhood conflicts is their inability to empathize or to identify with adolescents or their roles or to understand their needs. Instead, the parents' own unresolved conflicts and ambivalences are projected onto the child, recreating past conflicts emanating from the parents' families of origin. When this is the case, a child is covertly asked to enact a role in a parent's family drama. These kinds of expectations are extremely confusing to adolescents who are not aware that they have been placed in roles created by a parent's fantasy life; yet they wish to please their parents. Because it is important to please their parents in such subtle and double-bind situations, the adolescent concludes that he or she has committed some ill-defined wrongdoings. Under those circumstances, suicidal adolescents feel that they are a burden to their families and that everyone would be better off without them.

The Influence of the Social Factor on Adolescent Suicidal Behavior. The influential social factor on suicidal adolescent behavior is peer relationships. All adolescents struggle for acceptance in their peer group, which is a difficult task because of baffling requirements. However, suicidal adolescents generally do not feel accepted by normal peer groups. They are either loners or a member of an ostracized or non-accepted peer group. Many suicidal adolescents will establish close ties with much older young adults who are generally rejected by the adolescent's parents. Very often a suicidal gesture will be precipitated by the break up of a peer or love relationship. In these cases, acceptance has a life-or-death value. There are also adolescents who will do anything to be accepted by a peer group. These adolescents may either engage in delinquent behavior or substance abuse, or participate in dangerous rites, acts, or rituals at the price of self-contempt and hatred that may lead to a suicide attempt.

Treatment of the Suicidal Adolescent. The first task in treating the suicidal adolescent is to determine whether hospitalization is indicated. Some believe that all suicidal adolescents should be hospitalized for their own protection and to remove them from the painful environment (Marks, 1979). However, each case must be assessed and evaluated. Some criteria for recommending hospitalization are: (a) when the adolescent is psychotic, severely depressed, or unable to function; (b) when the family is uncooperative and refuses to participate in a treatment process; (c) when the family is unable or unwilling to provide sufficient environmental stability and protection for the child; and (d) when the adolescent has poor impulse control (Sands and Dixon, 1986). For those suicidal adolescents who are not hospitalized, treatment should proceed according to the crisis model. The adolescent and his or her family should be seen as soon as possible. The first task is to resolve the crippling effect of the crisis. The adolescent and each contributing family member should initially be seen separately and then together so the therapist can develop an accurate picture of family dynamics. The approach in the adolescent's individual session should be reality-oriented and logical, with the therapist making sure that the adolescent is encouraged to express painful feelings as well as those of anger and rage. The therapist should never say, "Think about what this is doing to your parents who love you." This is an insensitive statement that the adolescent really does not need since it only functions to reinforce feelings of rejection. The therapist should always stay where the client is when working individually with adolescents. In doing so the therapist will be sensitive to the ambivalence, scapegoat and double-binding tendencies that prevent the adolescent from establishing a close relationship (Sands and Dixon, 1986). Knowing this, the therapist must not force the relationship but should instead gently encourage it. In family treatment the therapist should focus on the cases of the precipitating problem and family pattern and functioning, especially marital interaction. The family is asked to face each other to discuss the precipitating problems and to share feelings and understanding. At the appropriate time, the therapist would help the family identify the nuclear problem. After the therapist has sufficient information about family functioning, the family should be helped to understand the different aspects of family functioning that contribute to the adolescent's suicidal behavior. Subsequent sessions should focus on the family's feelings about the causes of family dysfunctioning. This will lead to discussion of the marital problems. As the marital problems improve, so should family functioning.

After the crisis is over, the family should be referred for long-term treatment. Many professionals make the mistake of terminating treatment after the crisis is over. In cases of adolescent suicide, the problem is usually not resolved within the time constraints of the crisis period (Sands and Dixon, 1986). Personal and family conflicts can only be resolved by longer-term psychotherapy and family therapy.

By the conclusion of adolescence the young person should be accomplishing the task of separating from the parents, establishing an identity, preparing for a vocation, and deciding either to marry or remain single.

Young Adulthood

The time when young adulthood starts is not as discrete as in adolescence. It is generally established between the ages of 21 and 39. Some young people in college or graduate school who are financially dependent on their parents may experience a prolonged adolescence. In contrast, some teenagers who go to work immediately after high school graduation and live in their own apartments are functioning as adults. However, adulthood generally starts when the individual obtains a job and relative financial and emotional independence from his or her parents. Adequate psychosocial functioning and maturation are tasks of adulthood; development is the task of the childhood and adolescent years. Adequate psychosocial functioning is brought about by the integration of the experiences of the preceding years. It is facilitated by the relative absence of the influence of intrapsychic conflicts and the ability to use one's intelligence effectively. Adequately functioning adults accept reality that cannot be changed and, of course, change whatever in their best interests can be changed. They assume responsibility for themselves, a condition characterized by independence and self-control. They are able to express all emotions appropriately and are capable of giving and receiving love.

Work relationships and social relationships have specific values in the lives of young adults today. Young adults especially emphasize self-development, creativity, physical well-being, and self-fulfillment. They expect extensive rewards from their work such as good pay and high standards of living.

The new major tasks of young adulthood are the achievement of career goals, marriage, and parenthood. Although young people are getting married at a later age, at least 95 percent of all Americans will marry (Kaluger, 1979). Correspondingly, the divorce rate is variously estimated between 30 and 50 percent. It is clear that intimacy is a dominant struggle for today's young adults and is a major precipitant of crisis. Erikson (1968) identifies the crisis of young adulthood as being one of intimacy versus isolation.

The decisions made during young adulthood affect people throughout their lives. Decisions such as choice of occupation, marital status, and parenthood are made as a function of personality development.

Hence, they are an integral part of the ego and should be understood and evaluated from its perspective. The success of these decisions is determined by the stability of significant psychosocial needs existing at the time. When significant psychosocial needs change, whether they are needs for intimacy, ambition, prestige, or power, perceived ways of meeting them also change. We saw an example of this in the case of Mary, who married her husband because she had a need to be taken care of and protected from the cruel world. Her husband had a need to protect and care for her as a measure of his goodness and worth. Some 25 years later, her husband's needs changed and he divorced her because he wanted an independent, self-sufficient woman. Under such circumstances of crisis, it is important to understand personality development in order to understand the meaning of the crisis and to determine the most efficacious intervention method.

Middle Adulthood

The terms "middle adulthood," "middle life," and "middle age" are common terms used to describe the period of life from 40 to 65 years of age or the age of retirement. Middle adulthood is characterized by reaping what has been sown. It is the time of life when people become aware of mortality and the aging process. If the preceding years have been good—an evaluation often determined by occupational or economic success, a good marriage, and well-adjusted children—middle adulthood can be a very happy, problem-free time. People generally have more money and more free time, which provides them the opportunity to do things and enjoy love relationships more so than ever before. On the other hand, if the job, marriage, and children have not gone well, unhappiness and disappointment may characterize this phase of life. One's feelings can be dominated by the thought that it is too late to start over. Although there are specific physical changes and greater susceptibility to illness, psychological adjustment is much more important in terms of happiness for most people than is the effect of the actual physical changes.

Children can sometimes be a problem for married, middle-aged women. The problem, however, is not always the fact that the children move away from home but may also involve the return of children and grandchildren to the home.

Middle Adulthood Crisis. During young adulthood (21 to 40 years of age) most people function in a relatively stable and satisfactory manner, building over a period of some 20 years mechanisms to facilitate such functioning. Most have a family organization that has offered support and reinforcement. As individuals approach middle age, however, many of these stable conditions begin to change. It is the changes brought on by the human maturational process that make this phase of life potentially crisis producing. The first of these changes that a middle-aged individual must adapt to is the psychological awareness of aging. Signs of aging (balding, the need for bifocals, a tendency toward overweight, a greater propensity to tire, and a longer time to recover from illness) begin to show. Also, contemporaries begin to die, often unexpectedly of heart attacks. Certainly illness is more frequent. This awareness of the aging process causes the individual to become more conscious of self, resulting in a great deal of introspection and self-evaluation. The changes of middle life require adjustments. As we have seen, many middle-aged parents do not want this change. Changes in status or occupation can be another source of crisis. This was reflected in the case of John, who was transferred to Arizona after 24 years in the same city with the same company. The woman whose adult life has been spent raising a family is especially prone to middle-age crisis. In effect, she is forced into early retirement. For some women, menopause is a critical event, especially for those whose reproductive functions fulfilled multiple purposes. While there are physical discomforts associated with menopause, it is generally believed that they do not per se cause psychological debilitation. Neugarten (1975) did a cross-sectional study of menopause and concluded:

> This is not to say that the menopause is a meaningless phenomenon in the lives of women; nor that biological factors are of no importance in adult personality. Instead these comments are intended to point out: (1) that the menopause is not necessarily the important event in understanding the psychology of middle-aged women that we might have assumed it to be from a biological model or from psychoanalytic theory—not as important, seemingly, as illness, or even as worry over possible illness that might occur in one's husband rather than in oneself; (2) that the timing of the biological event, the climacterium—at least to the extent that we could perceive it—did not produce order in our data; and (3) above all, that psychologists should proceed cautiously in assuming the same intimate relationships between biological and psychological phenomenon in adulthood that hold true in childhood.

There have been some reports of menopause in men. If we consider the literal meaning of menopause, that is, the cessation of child-bearing capacity, there is no male menopause. However, some men may need to compensate for a feeling of sexual decline by either increasing their sexual activities or getting involved with other women. This situation often produces a crisis for the wife or the family more than for the individual, although a crisis can be produced by an individual's conflict over two loves. This was illustrated in the case of Rosemary (see chapter 2), whose husband Frank resolved his conflict by committing suicide.

In sum, middle age is more a state of mind than a physical change such as adolescence. Again, it is the reaction to the changes of middle age that produces a crisis.

A middle-age crisis can manifest itself in any of the ways that has been discussed thus far, in the individual or the family. Treatment proceeds on the same basis as set forth in chapter 5.

Late Adulthood (The Elderly)

Generally, age 65 or the age of retirement marks the beginning of late adulthood. The elderly are rapidly becoming a significant percentage (11 to 14 percent) of the American population, a youth-oriented culture.* The most salient characteristic of late adulthood is the retirement from work. Retirement means different things to different people. Some people look forward to it, seeing it as the opportunity to do the things they have planned for many years. Others whose egos were overly invested in their work may have a more difficult time. Still others will have a difficult time because of inadequate income, housing, or the inability to enjoy their free time with significant activities. There are also events that can make late adulthood a trying time; these include the prospect of the married person having to live alone, the fact that the children live in another city, the death of friends, and illness. The development of Alzheimers disease and other ailments associated with aging is also fairly common, and these conditions can cause enormous problems for the spouse or children.

The elderly must adapt to the decline of their authority and to the increase in their dependency on children or someone else. Erikson (1968) sees this phase as a choice between integrity and despair. Integrity means maintaining a sense of purpose and accomplishment, resulting in feelings of a life well lived. The major adaptive task is to find happiness and satisfaction.

Crises of the Elderly

At no other time in the life cycle does the human being have more to adjust to in order to maintain equilibrium than does the aged individual in the United States. First, the individual has to adjust to retirement and the loss of all the psychic values and benefits of an occupation; that is, status, self-esteem, and feelings of worth, as well as economic benefits. For many, this change is experienced as a loss. For others it is an eagerly awaited event that nevertheless requires a great deal of adjustment. The elderly individual has to adjust to physical changes, including a decrease in strength and an increase in illness. At some point there will probably

*From *Aging American—Trends and Projection* (1985–86), U.S. Department of Health and Human Services. Washington, D.C.: Author.

have to be an adjustment to the loss of a loved one, leaving the individual feeling alone and lonely. Consider the following case:

Mrs. Paulus, a 68-year-old widow, came to the crisis clinic to "get help with her depression." She was neatly dressed and very well groomed. Her posture was good with no motor retardation. There was no present sign of depression. She stated immediately that she was a great believer in therapy and that it had benefited several friends of hers. She specifically asked for a "compassionate, objective friend." She stated that she had never had psychiatric treatment before but now needed help to cope with this "aloneness and loneliness."

To adjust and maintain equilibrium, the aged person must be able to find a sense of self-worth. The individual may have to deal with a reversal of roles; for example, many elderly people become dependent on their children. Perhaps the aged person's greatest fear is not of death but of becoming dependent on children. All of these conditions tend to make the elderly feel afraid and confused. To counteract these feelings, they must have adequate coping mechanisms. When they do not, a crisis develops. Consider the following case:

Mrs. White, a 69-year-old woman, referred herself to the crisis center because she wanted help with her "ups and downs." She stated that she was "exceedingly low" today, since she was so worried about her daughter. She thought that she was trying to live her life through her daughter, and she came for help to "stop doing that."

Death of Spouse. The death of a spouse is a catastrophic event for everyone, but especially for the elderly. Gerber et al. (1975), Dimond (1981) and Sanders (1980) found that the elderly experienced more intense grief than younger spouses. Gerber (1975) found that normal grief reactions in the elderly are delayed or prolonged. The elderly generally have been married for 30 to 50 years, and the loss of a relationship of that duration is experienced as a significant one, regardless of the quality of the relationship. Certain roles and functions had been performed by both partners, and after a partner's death, the remaining partner must assume roles and functions never performed before. The adjustment to this event could affect the individual positively or negatively.

Interpersonal support can be a major factor in resolving a crisis in the elderly. Madison (1968) found that widows who had interpersonal support were doing well three months after the death of a spouse. Interpersonal support makes the elderly feel wanted and valuable. Family members, neighbors, and friends are a valuable source of support.

Treatment. Although the basic procedures set forth in chapter 5 apply to treating the aged, several variations are necessary for most effectiveness. First, it should be recognized that much of the elderly person's behavior is designed to counter the painful feelings of ego loss and impoverishment. Some of these coping mechanisms are constructive, others are not. They must be understood, including which ones are being used and how and the purpose they serve. The elderly person must be helped to counteract these feelings with constructive coping mechanisms. Second, intervention in the environment can sometimes aid this process. The major intervention technique with the aged should be psychological support. The focus should be on the individual's reaction to the stress or precipitating events causing the reaction. Third, the therapist should try to stimulate the individual's interest in social activities, especially those that enable the individual to be intellectually active. This may be difficult, however, for the elderly person who is depressed and feels hopeless. Fourth, as a person growths older, relatives and significant others are very important. Environmental support should be assessed and used at every opportunity.

Finally, the aged person should not be treated as a dependent child. The therapist's interaction should be one of respect and acceptance of the individual's capacity.

REFERENCES

Brenner, C. (1973). *An elementary textbook of psychoanalysis.* New York: International Universities Press.

Cosand, B. J., Bourque, L. B., & Kraus, J. F. (1982). Suicide adolescents in Sacramento county, CA, 1950—1979. *Adolescence, 17,* (68, Winter), 917–930.

Counts, R. M., & Sacks, A. (1985). The need for crisis intervention during marital separation. *Social Work, 30,* (2), 146–150.

Dimond, M. (1981). Bereavement and the elderly: A critical review with implications for nursing practice and research. *Journal of Advanced Nursing,* 6, 461–470.

Engel, G. L. (1962). *Psychological development in health and disease.* Philadelphia: W. B. Saunders.

Erikson, E. H. (1959). Growth and crisis of the health personality. In Identity and the life cycle: Selected papers [Monograph]. *Psychological Issues, 1,* (1), 50–100.

Erikson, E. H. (1963). *Childhood and society.* New York: W. W. Norton.

Erikson, E. H. (1968). *Identity, youth, and crisis.* New York: W. W. Norton.

Erikson, E. (1980). *Identity and the life cycle.* New York: W. W. Norton.

Gerber, I. et al. (1985). Anticipatory grief and aged widows and widowers. *Journal of Gerontology, 39,* (2), 225–229.

Goldstein, S., & Giddings, J. (1973). Multiple impact therapy: An approach to crisis intervention with families. In G. A. Spector, & W. L. Clarborn. (Eds.), *Crisis intervention.* New York: Behavioral Publications.

Holmes, T. H., & Rahe, R. H. (1967). The social readjustment rating scale. *Journal of Psychosomatic Research, 11,* (2), 213–218.

Kaluger, G., & Kaluger, M. F. (1979). *Human development* (2nd ed.). St. Louis: C. V. Mosby.

Madison, D., & Viola, A. (1968). The health of widows in the year following bereavement. *Journal of Psychosomatic Research, 12,* 297–306.

Mahler, M. S., Pine, F., & Bergman, A. (1975). *The psychological birth of the human infant.* New York: Basic Books, Inc.

Marks, A. (1979). Management of the suicidal adolescent on a nonpsychiatric adolescent unit. *Journal of Pediatrics, 95,* 305–308.

Neugarten, B. L. (1975). Adult personality: Toward a psychology of the life cycle. In W. Sze (Ed.), *Human life cycle.* New York: Jason Aronson.

Olsen, M. (1968). *The process of social organization.* New York: Holt, Rinehart and Winston.

Pfeffer, C. R. (1981). The family system of suicidal children. *American Journal of Psychotherapy, 35.*

Richman, J. J. (1971). Family determinants of suicide potential. In D. B. Anderson, & L. J. McClearn (Eds.), *Identifying suicide potential.* New York: Behavioral Publications.

Riskin, J. (1963). Methodology for studying family interaction. *Archives of General Psychiatry, 8,* 343–388.

Sanders, C. M. (1980–81). Comparison of younger and older spouses in bereavement outcome omega. *Journal of Death and Dying, 11,* (3), 217–232.

Sands, R. G., & Dixon, S. L. (1986). Adolescent crisis and suicidal behavior: Dynamics and treatment. *Child and Adolescent Social Work Journal, 3,* (2), 109–122.

Tishler, C. L., McKerny, P. C., & Morgan, K. C. (1981). Adolescent suicide attempts: Some significant factors. *Suicide and Life Threatening Behaviors, II,* (2, Spring), 86–92.

SUGGESTED READINGS

Ackerman, N. W. (1958). *The psychodynamics of family life: Diagnosis and treatment of family relationships.* New York: Basic Books.

Blos, P. (1970). *The young adolescent.* New York: The Free Press.

Butler, R. N., & Lewis, M. I. (1977). *Aging and mental health: Positive psychosocial approaches* (2nd ed.). St. Louis: C. V. Mosby.

Freud, A. (1975). Adolescence as a developmental disturbance. In W. Sze (Ed.), *Human life cycle* (pp. 245–250). New York: Jason Aronson. [Reprinted from G. Caplan & S. Lebovicis. (Eds.). (1969). *Adolescence: Psychosocial perspectives.* New York: Basic Books.]

Gitelson, M. (1948). The emotional problems of elderly persons. *Geriatrics, 3,*(3), 135–150.

Langsley, D. G., & Kapland, D. M. (Eds.). (1968). *The treatment of families in crisis.* New York: Grune & Stratton.

Peck, R. (1975). Psychological development in the second half of life. In W. Sze (Ed.), *Human life cycle.* New York: Jason Aronson.

Satir, V. M. (1964). *Conjoint family therapy: A guide to theory and teaching.* Palo Alto, Calif.: Science and Behavior Books.

Summary and Conclusion

This book provides a relatively comprehensive perspective of working with people in crisis, based on the premise that the more knowledge and understanding therapists have, the more effective they can be with skills and individual creativity. Accordingly, considerable focus is given to a functional definition of crisis and the premise of crisis theory. Since the natures of the social environment and the human being make perfect living impossible, states of upset are routine occurrences of everyday living. Hence one of the purposes of the socialization process is to prepare the individuals to adapt and cope with states of upset as they pursue personal happiness and life goals. It follows, therefore, that a crisis, as used in this book, is more than just being upset. It is being so overwhelmed with emotions that one is unable to function as effectively as before the crisis, and thus needs the assistance of another.

Since one cannot fail to function, the crisis therapist must intervene before ineffective functioning becomes a habitual pattern of dysfunctioning, commonly called psychopathology. Since the events that precipitate crises in some people are common problem-solving conditions for others, it is believed that a systematic approach to understanding human behavior will enable the crisis therapist to know why some people develop a crisis and others do not. Consequently, much emphasis is placed on the socialization process and psychic development. During the process of psychic development, adaptation patterns and specific forms of coping mechanisms are developed. These are discussed as an integral part of social functioning. To prepare the crisis therapist with the most important medium through which to apply knowledge and skills, communication theory and process are presented. This is the bridge between theory and techniques. The techniques of intervention presented are not limited to working with people in crisis, but are applicable to all therapeutic intervention. However, the crisis therapist must use them more rapidly and in a shorter period of time. In chapters 6 and 7, common reactions to crisis conditions are discussed in an effort to expand on the content in Part I. Some special crisis situations are presented; that is, suicidal behavior, homicidal behavior, and rape. The final chapter touches on the family in crisis and on the common life crises of adolescence, middle age, and old age.

It is my hope that the contents of this book will contribute to enhancing the knowledge, skill, and effectiveness of those who work with people in crisis. More important, I hope that a comprehensive approach to the individual in crisis will result in more than a "stop for first aid" philosophy that characterizes current crisis theory. Although the temporal limits of crisis theory can be followed, the crisis therapist should devote time and research to learning to do as much as possible to strengthen and resolidify the functioning of the individual in crisis. It is believed that crisis treatment can move beyond the goal of restoring the individual to a precrisis level of functioning.

Name Index

Subject Index

Subject Index